FIREFLY•POCKET•GUIDES

SKELETONS

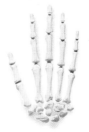

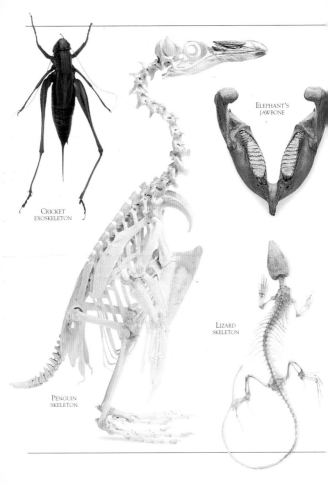

CRICKET
EXOSKELETON

ELEPHANT'S
JAWBONE

LIZARD
SKELETON

PENGUIN
SKELETON

FIREFLY · POCKET · GUIDES

SKELETONS

Written by
BARBARA TAYLOR

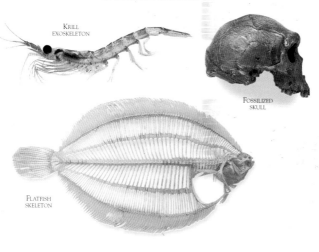

KRILL
EXOSKELETON

FOSSILIZED
SKULL

FLATFISH
SKELETON

FIREFLY BOOKS

A DK PUBLISHING BOOK

Project directors	Bob Gordon, Helen Parker
Editor	Neil Kelly
Art editor	Thomas Keenes
DK team	Jane Yorke, Marcus James
Production	Joanne Rooke
Picture research	Caroline Allen, Christine Rista
Jacket design	Dean Price
US editors	Jennifer Dorr, William Lach

First published in Canada in 1998
by Firefly Books Ltd.
3680 Victoria Park Avenue,
Willowdale, Ontario, Canada
M2H 3K1

Canadian Cataloguing in Publication Data

Taylor, Barbara, 1954–
  Skeletons

(Firefly pocket guides)
Includes index.
ISBN 1-55209-248-8

1. Skeleton. 2. Bones. I. Title. II. Series.

QL821.T39 1998   573.7'6   C97-932699-0

Color reproduction by Colourscan, Singapore
Printed and bound in Italy by L.E.G.O.

CONTENTS

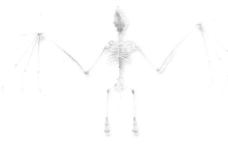

How to use this book 8

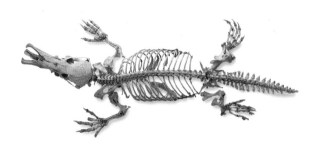

How to use this book

These pages show you how to use *Firefly Pocket Guides: Skeletons*. Each of the six sections of the book opens with a double-page picture. There is an introductory section at the front and a reference section at the back. The four main sections look at the human skeleton, internal and external skeletons, and fossilized skeletons.

HEADING AND INTRODUCTION
This provides a clear overview of the subject. After reading this, you should have an idea what the pages are about. This page is about echinoderms and mollusks, and is found in the Skeletons on the Outside section.

CORNER CODING
The corners of the pages in each section are color-coded as follows to remind you which section you are in.

■ HUMAN SKELETON

■ SKELETONS ON THE INSIDE

■ SKELETONS ON THE OUTSIDE

■ ANCIENT SKELETONS

Corner coding

Heading

Introduction

Annotation

Caption

Label

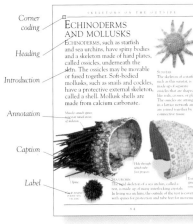

ECHINODERMS AND MOLLUSKS
ECHINODERMS, such as starfish and sea urchins, have spiny bodies and a skeleton made of hard plates, called ossicles, underneath the skin. The ossicles may be movable or fused together. Soft-bodied mollusks, such as snails and cockles, have a protective external skeleton, called a shell. Mollusk shells are made from calcium carbonate.

SEA STAR
The skeleton of a starfish such as this sunstar, is made up of separate ossicles that are shaped like rods, crosses, or plates. The ossicles are arranged in a lattice network that are joined together by connective tissue.

Muscles attach plates to rest of raised areas of skeleton

Hole through which tube feet protrude

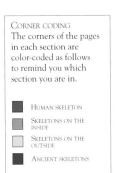

Spine

SEA URCHINS
The rigid skeleton of a sea urchin, called a test, is made up of many interlocking crystals. In living sea urchins, the outside of the skeleton is covered with spines for protection and tube feet for movement.

CAPTIONS
Each illustration, whether an artwork, a photograph, or a diagram, is accompanied by an explanatory caption.

LABELS
Some pictures have labels. These give extra information about the picture or may provide clearer identification.

RUNNING HEADS
These remind you which section of the book you are in. The running head at the top of the left-hand page gives the section. The running head at the top of the right-hand page gives the subject.

FACT BOXES
Some pages have fact boxes. These contain at-a-glance information on the subject. This fact box gives details about the largest land snail and the feeding habits of the *Euglandina* snail.

LIFE ILLUSTRATION
Many of the skeletons in this book have an illustration to show what the animal looked like when it was alive.

Running head   *Fact box*

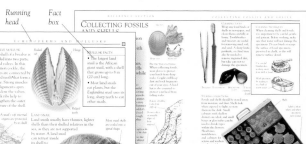

COLLECTING FOSSILS AND SHELLS

MOLLUSC FACTS
• The largest land snail is the African giant snail, with a shell that grows up to 39 cm (15 in) long.
• Most land snails eat plants, but the *Euglandina* snail uses its long, sharp teeth to eat other snails.

ECHINODERMS AND MOLLUSCS

BIVALVE MOLLUSC
The shell of a bivalve is divided into two parts, called valves. In this common cockle, the valves are connected by ridged teeth that form a hinge. Strong muscles and ligaments open and close the valves. Thick ribs help to strengthen the outer structure of the shell.

A snail's soft internal organs are protected by its shell

LAND SNAIL
Land snails usually have thinner, lighter shells than their shelled relatives in the sea, as they are not supported by water. A land snail can retreat inside its shell to escape danger or to survive cold or dry weather.

Most snail shells are coiled into a spiral shape

Tentacle
Eye
Head
Foot

Spaces filled with gas or fluid

CUTTLEFISH

CUTTLEFISH
A cuttlefish "bone" is in fact the animal's internal shell. The cuttlefish controls its movement by filling the many spaces in the shell with gas to make it rise, or fluid to make it sink.

Life illustration

REFERENCE SECTION
The reference pages are yellow and appear at the back of the book. On these, you will find useful facts, figures, and advice. These pages include skeleton records and tips on collecting bones, fossils, and shells.

ANNOTATION
Styled in *italics*, annotation points out noteworthy features of an illustration or photograph. It is usually accompanied by a leader line and often gives extra information.

GLOSSARY AND INDEX
At the back of the book is a glossary, which defines some of the terms used in the book. This is followed by an index, for quick reference to each subject.

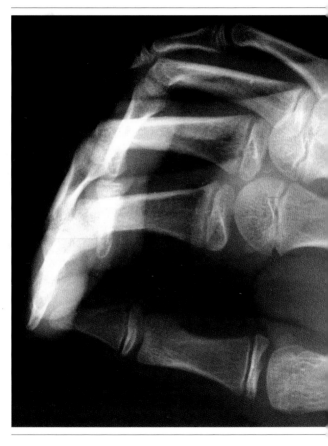

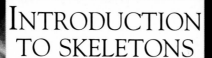

INTRODUCTION TO SKELETONS

WHAT IS A SKELETON?

A SKELETON IS a strong framework that supports and protects an animal's body. In many animals, the skeleton helps with movement as well. Most animals have either a skeleton on the inside of the body (endoskeleton) or a skeleton on the outside (exoskeleton), but some animals have both. A skeleton is usually made of hard materials, such as bone or chitin.

Bony tail club (see p. 103)

EUOPLOCEPHALUS

Spinal column (backbone)

WATER SUPPORT
A jellyfish does not have a skeleton because its body, which is 95 percent water, is supported by the water it lives in. Out of the water, its body collapses and is shapeless.

Exoskeleton

Jointed, flexible legs for movement

Pelvis (hipbones)

Caudal (tail) vertebrae

Patella (kneecap)

EXOSKELETONS
Most animals without backbones (invertebrates) have an exoskeleton. Like internal skeletons, these hard outer casings give an animal its shape and provide support and protection.

Foot bones form part of legs (see p. 36)

Two weight-bearing toes on each foot (see p. 60)

WOOD-BORING BEETLE

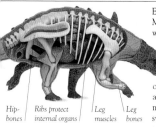

ENDOSKELETON MOVEMENT

Most endoskeletons are made up of bones, with muscles attached to them. The muscles contract to pull the bones into different positions, enabling an animal to move. The dinosaur *Euoplocephalus* had broad hipbones and fused spines on its backbone, which anchored the muscles that moved its back legs and swung the heavy tail.

Hip-bones

Ribs protect internal organs

Leg muscles

Leg bones

Horn *(see p. 28)*

Cervical (neck) vertebrae

Skull *(see p. 22)*

Orbit (eye socket)

Nasal (nose) bone

Molar (grinding) teeth

Jawbone *(see p. 24)*

Strong ribs

Elbow joint *(see p. 32)*

CHILLINGHAM BULL

ENDOSKELETONS

The spinal column of a vertebrate (an animal with a backbone) supports the body and the main parts of the endoskeleton. The skull, located at the top of the backbone, protects the brain. The ribs project from the sides of the backbone, as do the bones and cartilage that support the animal's limbs, wings, or fins.

Types of animal skeletons

Animal skeletons come in a variety of different shapes and sizes. As well as the bony endoskeletons of vertebrates, there are also the external shells of mollusks, such as snails and clams, the spiny exoskeletons of echinoderms, such as starfish and sea urchins, and the tough cases of arthropods, such as insects and spiders. Even worms have a fluid-filled, or hydrostatic, skeleton.

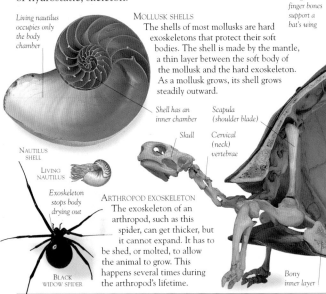

Long, thin finger bones support a bat's wing

Living nautilus occupies only the body chamber

MOLLUSK SHELLS
The shells of most mollusks are hard exoskeletons that protect their soft bodies. The shell is made by the mantle, a thin layer between the soft body of the mollusk and the hard exoskeleton. As a mollusk grows, its shell grows steadily outward.

Shell has an inner chamber

Scapula (shoulder blade)

Skull

Cervical (neck) vertebrae

NAUTILUS SHELL

LIVING NAUTILUS

Exoskeleton stops body drying out

ARTHROPOD EXOSKELETON
The exoskeleton of an arthropod, such as this spider, can get thicker, but it cannot expand. It has to be shed, or molted, to allow the animal to grow. This happens several times during the arthropod's lifetime.

BLACK WIDOW SPIDER

Bony inner layer

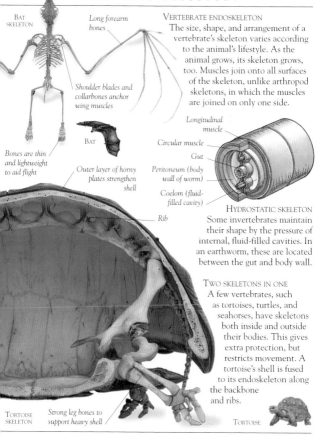

BAT SKELETON

Long forearm bones

Shoulder blades and collarbones anchor wing muscles

BAT

Bones are thin and lightweight to aid flight

Outer layer of horny plates strengthen shell

Rib

TORTOISE SKELETON

Strong leg bones to support heavy shell

TORTOISE

VERTEBRATE ENDOSKELETON

The size, shape, and arrangement of a vertebrate's skeleton varies according to the animal's lifestyle. As the animal grows, its skeleton grows, too. Muscles join onto all surfaces of the skeleton, unlike arthropod skeletons, in which the muscles are joined on only one side.

Longitudinal muscle

Circular muscle

Gut

Peritoneum (body wall of worm)

Coelom (fluid-filled cavity)

HYDROSTATIC SKELETON

Some invertebrates maintain their shape by the pressure of internal, fluid-filled cavities. In an earthworm, these are located between the gut and body wall.

TWO SKELETONS IN ONE

A few vertebrates, such as tortoises, turtles, and seahorses, have skeletons both inside and outside their bodies. This gives extra protection, but restricts movement. A tortoise's shell is fused to its endoskeleton along the backbone and ribs.

WHAT ARE SKELETONS MADE OF?

THE SKELETON OF a vertebrate is made mainly of bone and cartilage (gristle). Both are strong materials, but cartilage is more flexible than bone. Invertebrate skeletons are made mainly of materials such as chitin (in arthropods) and calcium carbonate (in mollusks).

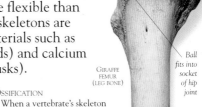

Giraffe thighbones are very long; this bone is 1 ft 9 in (52 cm) long

GIRAFFE FEMUR (LEG BONE)

Ball fits into socket of hip joint

Shaft bears weight of body

Lower limb bones fit here

HUMAN FETUS

OSSIFICATION

When a vertebrate's skeleton first forms, it is made of tough, rubbery cartilage. As the fetus develops, mineral salts and protein fibers are secreted into the cartilage, which gradually hardens, or ossifies, into bone.

Skeletal tissue is stained red to show ossification; cartilage remains white

BONE

Bone is a strong, slightly flexible substance. Its lightweight structure is composed of water, mineral salts, and collagen.

Ossification of leg tissue begins at six to 12 weeks

SHELL STRUCTURE

An animal's exoskeleton, or shell, may be formed from one or several substances. A tortoise's shell is made up of bony plates covered in keratin. Snail shells and seashells (such as this scallop shell) are made from calcium carbonate, while arthropod shells are made mainly of chitin.

SCALLOP SHELL

A scallop shell is divided into two halves

Epicuticle (nonchitinous outer layer)

Chitinous sensory hair, or seta

Ribs provide strength

Procuticle (chitinous inner layer)

Epidermal cells

BLACK RHINO HORN

Matted hair fibers

HAIRY HORN

Horn is composed of many compressed hair fibers. Hair is made from the structural protein keratin, which also forms nails and feathers. Unlike horns, antlers, such as those of a deer, are made entirely from bone.

CHITINOUS CUTICLE

Chitin is a substance found in the outer layer (cuticle) of the exoskeletons of insects, spiders, scorpions, and other arthropods. Its crisscrossed, layered structure makes it light and extra strong.

SILICA SKELETONS

Diatoms are microscopic, single-celled algae with skeletons formed from silica. The two halves of a diatom skeleton fit neatly together, like a box and its lid. Diatoms come in a great variety of shapes and are marked with delicate patterns.

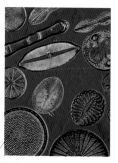

Frustule (Silica shell)

Skull bone

BONE

LIVING BONE is a growing substance that can repair itself when damaged. Bone constantly remodels itself, with osteoblast cells making new bone, and osteoclast cells breaking down old bone. Most bones have a smooth outer layer of solid, compact bone and an inner layer of light, spongy (cancellous) bone.

Lamella

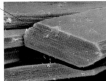

LAMELLAE
Compact bone is made up of tiny tubes called osteons. An osteon consists of lamellae (concentric layers) composed of collagen fibers and mineral salts, which surround a central canal for blood vessels and nerves.

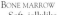

BONE MARROW
Soft, jellylike marrow fills the spaces in the middle of many bones. Red marrow makes red and white blood cells, which are carried into the bloodstream by blood vessels. Yellow marrow stores fat.

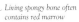

Living spongy bone often contains red marrow

BONE STRUCTURE
A living bone, such as this femur (thigh bone), has several layers. Wrapped around the outside of the bone is a thin, skinlike membrane called the periosteum, which contains nerves and blood vessels. The solid knob or head at the end of a bone is made of spongy bone.

HUMAN BREASTBONE

Head of bone

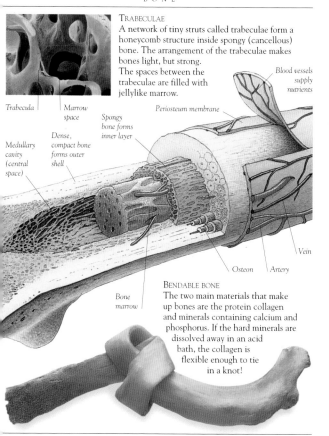

TRABECULAE

A network of tiny struts called trabeculae form a honeycomb structure inside spongy (cancellous) bone. The arrangement of the trabeculae makes bones light, but strong. The spaces between the trabeculae are filled with jellylike marrow.

Blood vessels supply nutrients

Trabecula

Marrow space

Spongy bone forms inner layer

Periosteum membrane

Medullary cavity (central space)

Dense, compact bone forms outer shell

Vein

Osteon *Artery*

Bone marrow

BENDABLE BONE

The two main materials that make up bones are the protein collagen and minerals containing calcium and phosphorus. If the hard minerals are dissolved away in an acid bath, the collagen is flexible enough to tie in a knot!

Repairing and replacing bones

If bones are cracked or broken (fractured), they can usually mend themselves. Some broken bones need to be held in place so that the bones knit together properly as they heal. This can be done with a splint, traction, a plaster of Paris cast, or internal splints made from metal.

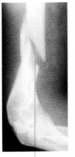 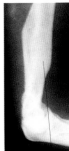

BROKEN ARM
These X-ray photographs of a human humerus (upper arm bone) show how effectively the body can heal broken bones. The time the bone takes to mend depends on the complexity or severity of the break.

Fractured bone on day of break

Several months later, bone has healed perfectly

NATURAL HEALING

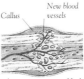

Clot of blood

Marrow   Torn blood vessels

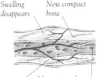

Callus   New blood vessels   Swelling disappears   New compact bone

Healed fracture   New spongy bone

1 UNLUCKY BREAK
When a bone breaks, blood from damaged vessels in the bone marrow forms a large clot around the fracture.

2 HEALING PROCESS
Collagen fibers start to join up the broken ends of bone. Repair tissues form a protective swelling (callus) around the break.

3 REPAIRED BONE
New bone fills the break. Spongy bone replaces repair tissue. Compact bone forms around the outer edge.

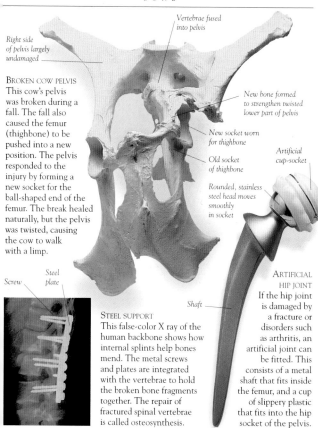

Right side of pelvis largely undamaged

Vertebrae fused into pelvis

New bone formed to strengthen twisted lower part of pelvis

New socket worn for thighbone

Old socket of thighbone

Artificial cup-socket

Rounded, stainless steel head moves smoothly in socket

BROKEN COW PELVIS
This cow's pelvis was broken during a fall. The fall also caused the femur (thighbone) to be pushed into a new position. The pelvis responded to the injury by forming a new socket for the ball-shaped end of the femur. The break healed naturally, but the pelvis was twisted, causing the cow to walk with a limp.

Screw

Steel plate

Shaft

ARTIFICIAL HIP JOINT
If the hip joint is damaged by a fracture or disorders such as arthritis, an artificial joint can be fitted. This consists of a metal shaft that fits inside the femur, and a cup of slippery plastic that fits into the hip socket of the pelvis.

STEEL SUPPORT
This false-color X ray of the human backbone shows how internal splints help bones mend. The metal screws and plates are integrated with the vertebrae to hold the broken bone fragments together. The repair of fractured spinal vertebrae is called osteosynthesis.

SKULLS AND SENSES

AN ANIMAL'S SKULL is a hard, bony case that protects the brain and sense organs. Skull adaptations, including toothed jaws, beaks, bills, and snouts, enable different animals to feed in a variety of ways. In some animals, such as dogs, the braincase, or cranium, has a bony ridge on top to anchor the jaw muscles.

Large brain cavity

Higher right ear cavity

Nasal passage

Roof of mouth

BABOON SKULL
This cross section of a baboon's skull shows the bony cavities that protect the brain, eyes, organs of smell, and the tongue. The inner ear bones are hidden deep inside the skull.

Lower left ear cavity

Binocular vision

Monocular vision (right eye only)

OWL SKULL, TOP VIEW

OWL SKULL
An owl's ears are often at different levels in the skull. Each ear catches sounds at a slightly different time, enabling the owl to pinpoint the direction of its prey with great accuracy.

Monocular vision (left eye only)

WOODCOCK SKULL, TOP VIEW

BIRD VISION
The eyes of most predatory birds, such as owls, point directly forward. This gives a wide field of binocular (two-eyed) vision. Birds that are hunted, such as woodcock, tend to have eyes that point in opposite directions. This enables them to look for danger all around and above, without moving their head.

Forward binocular vision *Monocular vision* *Blind spot* *Rear binocular vision*

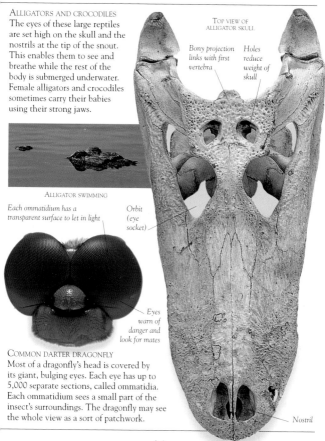

ALLIGATORS AND CROCODILES
The eyes of these large reptiles are set high on the skull and the nostrils at the tip of the snout. This enables them to see and breathe while the rest of the body is submerged underwater. Female alligators and crocodiles sometimes carry their babies using their strong jaws.

TOP VIEW OF ALLIGATOR SKULL

Bony projection links with first vertebra

Holes reduce weight of skull

ALLIGATOR SWIMMING

Each ommatidium has a transparent surface to let in light

Orbit (eye socket)

Eyes warn of danger and look for mates

COMMON DARTER DRAGONFLY
Most of a dragonfly's head is covered by its giant, bulging eyes. Each eye has up to 5,000 separate sections, called ommatidia. Each ommatidium sees a small part of the insect's surroundings. The dragonfly may see the whole view as a sort of patchwork.

Nostril

23

TEETH AND JAWS

ANIMALS USE their teeth and jaws for catching prey, cutting and grinding up food, and for defense. An animal's teeth and jaw shape vary depending on whether it is a plant-eater (herbivore), meat-eater (carnivore), or eater of both plants and meat (omnivore).

Enamel layer

Dentine

Blood vessels and nerves in pulp cavity

Gum

Jawbone

Blood vessels and nerves

TOOTH STRUCTURE
The outer layer of a tooth is made of enamel, the hardest substance that the body can produce. Inside the enamel is a layer of tough dentine, which cushions the tooth against knocks and blows. The pulp cavity in the middle of the tooth contains nerves and blood vessels.

TYPES OF TEETH
Mammal teeth are shaped for different functions. A dog uses its incisor and canine teeth to seize food, which is then sliced up by the carnassial teeth. The molar and premolars chew the food for swallowing.

Incisor

Molar *Carnassial* *Premolar*

DOG'S TEETH

Canine

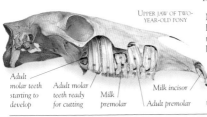

UPPER JAW OF TWO-
YEAR-OLD PONY

Adult molar teeth starting to develop

Adult molar teeth ready for cutting

Milk premolar

Milk incisor

Adult premolar

MILK AND ADULT TEETH
Like all mammals, horses have two sets of teeth. Milk, or baby, teeth erupt through the jawbones first. These are later replaced by adult, or permanent, teeth, which gradually wear down throughout the horse's life.

HERBIVORE

Plant-eaters, such as this goat, have a deep lower jawbone to anchor the large, strong chewing muscle. Most of the teeth are grinding molars at the back of the mouth. A goat has no top front teeth.

GOAT SKULL

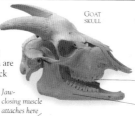

Lower jaw moves from side to side and back and forth.

Jaw-closing muscle attaches here

Molar and premolar teeth

Deep lower jaw for muscle attachment

CARNIVORE

Most meat-eaters have thick, heavy jaws, with a flange at the back of the skull for attachment of the powerful jaw-closing muscle. A lion has a massive cheek ridge, which anchors its strong lower jaw muscle.

LION SKULL

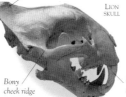

Lower jaw moves up and down only.

Bony cheek ridge

Canines seize and tear prey

OMNIVORE

Animals that eat both plants and meat have less specialized teeth. A chimp's teeth mainly slice and chew, as it uses its hands to gather food. As its rigid jaw has limited sideways movement, a chimp's teeth are worn into points and cusps.

CHIMPANZEE SKULL

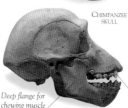

Lower jaw moves up and down.

Limited sideways movement.

Deep flange for chewing muscle

Large canines

RODENT

All rodents, such as squirrels and coypus, are herbivores, but their four, large front teeth are adapted for gnawing. These teeth are worn down by use, but never stop growing.

COYPU SKULL

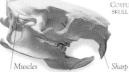

Lower jaw moves up and down.

Muscles attach here

Sharp gnawing teeth

SPECIALIZED MOUTHPARTS

ANIMALS ARE adapted for feeding in a variety of
ways. Some animals gather food using specialized
mouthparts, such as beaks, snouts, feeding
tubes, and slicing mandibles.

Cranium

Long nasal bone   *Mandible*

*Orbit
(eye
socket)*   *Ear
cavity*

GIANT ANTEATER
As they have no teeth, giant anteaters rely on their probing snout
and long, sticky tongue to trap insects such as ants and termites.
Horny projections in the mouth and muscular stomach mash up food.

BIRDS' BEAKS
Instead of a heavy jawbone, jaw muscles, and
teeth, birds have a lightweight, toothless,
horny beak. Also called a bill, the shape and
size of the mouthpart varies greatly, allowing
different birds to tackle a wide range of foods.
Birds grind up food in a muscular
part of the stomach, called the
gizzard. Plant-eating birds may
swallow grit to aid digestion.

*Cone-shaped
bill*

FINCH SKULL   SEEDS

*Chisel-like
beak*

MEAT   WOODPECKER SKULL   INSECTS AND
ARTHROPODS

KESTREL SKULL

*Hooked beak
to tear up food*

JAY SKULL

*Strong, all-
purpose bill*

CHEWING THROAT

The common European bream has a "pouting" mouth, which it uses to suck up worms, insect larvae, and mollusks. These are then ground up by the pharyngeal teeth, which are located inside the throat.

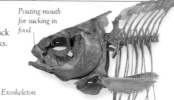

Pouting mouth for sucking in food

Exoskeleton

MOVABLE JAW

Sea urchins chew their food with a five-toothed jaw made up of bony plates. The jaw is often referred to as "Aristotle's lantern" because it resembles an old oil lamp. Muscles open and close the bony plates and push and pull the jaw structure in and out of the urchin's mouth.

"Aristotle's lantern" on underside of urchin, facing seabed

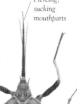

Piercing, sucking mouthparts

Proboscis, can be coiled up when not in use

Powerful, jawlike mandibles

WASP FEEDING

A wasp has sharp-edged mandibles for cutting, tearing, and crushing. It also has a short, broad tongue to lap up liquids.

BUTTERFLY'S PROBOSCIS

Adult butterflies suck up food through a long tube called a proboscis, which is made from two joined-up mouthparts.

BLOODSUCKING FLY

The tabanid fly uses its needlelike mouthpart to pierce a victim's skin. The other mouthparts form a tube to suck up the blood.

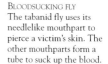

TUSKS, HORNS, AND ANTLERS

MANY MAMMALS have long, pointed structures that project from their skulls; these are used for self-defense or for fighting with rival animals of the same kind for mates. These structures include the tusks of walruses, elephants, and narwhals, the horns of rhinos or antelope, and the antlers of elk and deer.

Heavy skull used to smash through thick ice to make breathing holes

Tusklike teeth

Tusks continue to grow throughout life

LONG IN THE TOOTH
The upper canine teeth of a walrus grow into tusks up to 3 ft (1 m) long. Tusk size determines a walrus's social status within a group. Male walruses have bigger, heavier tusks than females.

MUNTJAC SKULL
A male muntjac deer has short, pointed antlers and two large, tusklike canine teeth in its upper jaw. When rival bucks (males) battle to win mating rights over a group of does (females), they use their "tusks" rather than their antlers.

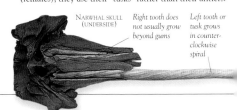

NARWHAL SKULL
(UNDERSIDE)

Right tooth does not usually grow beyond gums

Left tooth or tusk grows in counterclockwise spiral

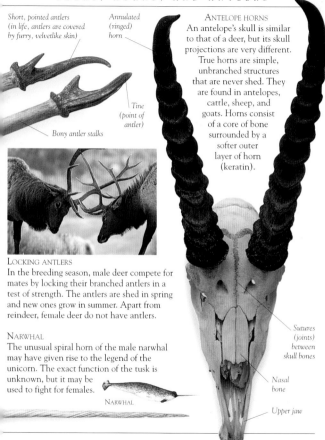

Short, pointed antlers (in life, antlers are covered by furry, velvetlike skin)

Annulated (ringed) horn

Tine (point of antler)

Bony antler stalks

ANTELOPE HORNS

An antelope's skull is similar to that of a deer, but its skull projections are very different. True horns are simple, unbranched structures that are never shed. They are found in antelopes, cattle, sheep, and goats. Horns consist of a core of bone surrounded by a softer outer layer of horn (keratin).

LOCKING ANTLERS

In the breeding season, male deer compete for mates by locking their branched antlers in a test of strength. The antlers are shed in spring and new ones grow in summer. Apart from reindeer, female deer do not have antlers.

NARWHAL

The unusual spiral horn of the male narwhal may have given rise to the legend of the unicorn. The exact function of the tusk is unknown, but it may be used to fight for females.

NARWHAL

Sutures (joints) between skull bones

Nasal bone

Upper jaw

SKELETONS FOR DEFENSE

LIKE SUITS OF ARMOR, exoskeletons, such as shells or hard wing cases, can protect animals from predators. Many exoskeletons are patterned, colored, or disguised to deter would-be attackers. Some endoskeletons have special defensive features, such as spines or blades.

Colors and stripes warn off attackers

Spines

LIONFISH

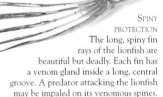

A yellow, red, or black exoskeleton indicates danger

Needle-sharp spines are filled with poison

Base of fin rays

WARNING COLORS

Many insects, such as this shieldbug, have colored or patterned casings to warn predators that they are poisonous or taste unpleasant. When attacked, this shieldbug gives off a foul-smelling liquid.

SPINY PROTECTION

The long, spiny fin rays of the lionfish are beautiful but deadly. Each fin has a venom gland inside a long, central groove. A predator attacking the lionfish may be impaled on its venomous spines.

CAMOUFLAGED EXOSKELETON

This leaf insect's disguised exoskeleton enables it to hide from predators. The leaflike camouflage works best if the insect keeps perfectly still, as the slightest movement could give away its position.

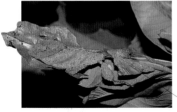

Leaf insect blends into its surroundings for protection

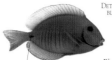

DETAIL OF
BLADE

*Lancet blade cuts flesh
like a surgeon's scalpel*

*Blade
extends
at right angles*

SURGEONFISH

The surgeonfish is named for its
bony, razor-sharp "lancet" blade
on either side of its body, near
the base of the tail. When
attacked, the surgeonfish
thrashes its tail at the predator,
inflicting terrible wounds.

BREAKAWAY
If grabbed by a predator, most lizards
can quickly shed their tail and escape.
The shed tail often twitches after it
has been severed, confusing
the attacker while the lizard gets
away. Fracture points along the
tail vertebrae mark the
points where the tail
can break off.

*Tail (caudal)
vertebrae*

*Fracture
points*

LIZARD TAIL
BONES

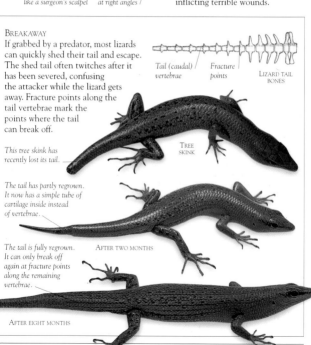

*This tree skink has
recently lost its tail.*

TREE
SKINK

*The tail has partly regrown.
It now has a simple tube of
cartilage inside instead
of vertebrae.*

*The tail is fully regrown.
It can only break off
again at fracture points
along the remaining
vertebrae.*

AFTER TWO MONTHS

AFTER EIGHT MONTHS

JOINTS AND MOVEMENT

JOINTS ARE LOCATED where the inflexible parts of a skeleton, such as the hard bones of an endoskeleton or the tough plates of an exoskeleton, come into contact. Exoskeleton joints are fairly flexible, but some endoskeleton joints are fixed or only partly movable.

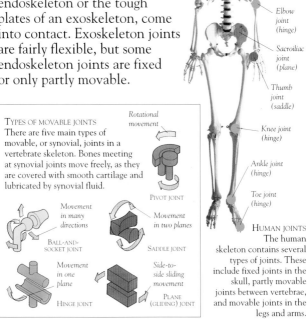

Intervertebral joint (pivot)

Shoulder joint (ball-and-socket)

Vertebrocostal joint (plane)

Elbow joint (hinge)

Sacroiliac joint (plane)

Thumb joint (saddle)

Knee joint (hinge)

Ankle joint (hinge)

Toe joint (hinge)

TYPES OF MOVABLE JOINTS
There are five main types of movable, or synovial, joints in a vertebrate skeleton. Bones meeting at synovial joints move freely, as they are covered with smooth cartilage and lubricated by synovial fluid.

Rotational movement

PIVOT JOINT

Movement in many directions

BALL-AND-SOCKET JOINT

Movement in two planes

SADDLE JOINT

Movement in one plane

HINGE JOINT

Side-to-side sliding movement

PLANE (GLIDING) JOINT

HUMAN JOINTS
The human skeleton contains several types of joints. These include fixed joints in the skull, partly movable joints between vertebrae, and movable joints in the legs and arms.

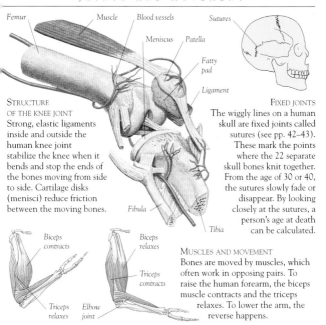

STRUCTURE OF THE KNEE JOINT

Strong, elastic ligaments inside and outside the human knee joint stabilize the knee when it bends and stop the ends of the bones moving from side to side. Cartilage disks (menisci) reduce friction between the moving bones.

Femur
Muscle
Blood vessels
Meniscus
Patella
Fatty pad
Ligament
Fibula
Tibia

FIXED JOINTS

The wiggly lines on a human skull are fixed joints called sutures (see pp. 42–43). These mark the points where the 22 separate skull bones knit together. From the age of 30 or 40, the sutures slowly fade or disappear. By looking closely at the sutures, a person's age at death can be calculated.

Sutures

MUSCLES AND MOVEMENT

Bones are moved by muscles, which often work in opposing pairs. To raise the human forearm, the biceps muscle contracts and the triceps relaxes. To lower the arm, the reverse happens.

Biceps contracts
Triceps relaxes
Biceps relaxes
Triceps contracts
Elbow joint

WALKING MECHANISM IN AN INSECT

The hard plates that make up an insect exoskeleton meet at flexible joints. Muscles, attached to the exoskeleton across these joints, contract to produce walking movement.

Protractor muscle pulls limb forward
Retractor muscle pulls limb backward
Extensor muscle pulls limb upward
Joint
Flexor muscle pulls limb downward
Limb

Arms, wings, and flippers

Vertebrate forelimbs are adapted for different functions. Some vertebrates have arms, which are used for walking, feeding, or hanging. Others have wings for flying or flippers for swimming. Different types of forelimbs are often made up of similar bones but vary in the number, size, and shape of the bones. Invertebrate forelimbs also vary in size, shape, and function.

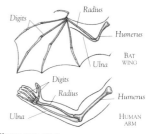

Digits
Radius
Humerus
Ulna
BAT WING

Digits
Radius
Humerus
Ulna
HUMAN ARM

WINGS AND ARMS

A bat's wing and a human forelimb are adapted for different purposes, but both are built from the same sets of bones. Bats have long finger bones to form the wings, while humans have large arm bones adapted for carrying heavy loads.

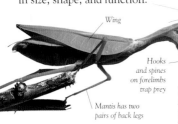

Wing

Hooks and spines on forelimbs trap prey

Mantis has two pairs of back legs

Grasping forelimb

Fly caught by mantis

PRAYING MANTIS

A mantis uses its strong, spiny forelimbs to catch insects. The mantis lies in wait for its prey and then shoots its forelimbs forward at great speed. The spines snap shut around the prey, holding it firmly as the mantis begins to eat it.

WINGED RAY

Rays have wide, winglike pectoral fins. They "fly" through the water by waving the edges of their fins. The up-and-down movement creates a wave that pushes the ray along. The whiplike tail provides little pushing power.

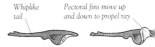

Whiplike tail

Pectoral fins move up and down to propel ray

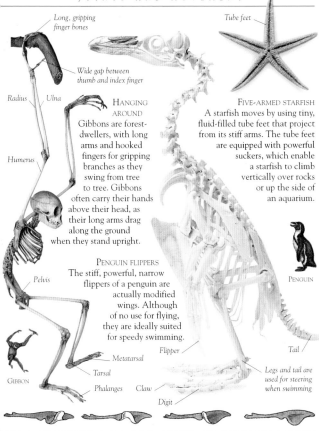

Long, gripping
finger bones

Wide gap between
thumb and index finger

Radius   Ulna

Humerus

Tube feet

HANGING AROUND
Gibbons are forest-dwellers, with long arms and hooked fingers for gripping branches as they swing from tree to tree. Gibbons often carry their hands above their head, as their long arms drag along the ground when they stand upright.

FIVE-ARMED STARFISH
A starfish moves by using tiny, fluid-filled tube feet that project from its stiff arms. The tube feet are equipped with powerful suckers, which enable a starfish to climb vertically over rocks or up the side of an aquarium.

PENGUIN FLIPPERS
The stiff, powerful, narrow flippers of a penguin are actually modified wings. Although of no use for flying, they are ideally suited for speedy swimming.

Pelvis

PENGUIN

Metatarsal

Tarsal

GIBBON

Phalanges

Flipper

Claw

Digit

Tail

Legs and tail are used for steering when swimming

Legs, feet, and tails

Back limbs are usually more powerful than
forelimbs and provide most of the force
needed for walking, running, and jumping.
They can also be used for digging and
grooming. On land, tails are used for balance
or for clinging to branches, but in water they
are often used for propulsion.

Backward-pointing spines

Fused lower limb bones

FLEA

A flea has powerful back legs
that enable it to jump more
than 12 in (30 cm) through
the air. While living on the
body of its host, a flea usually
moves around by walking.
Strong claws grip the host's hairs
or feathers, while pointed spines
covering the flea's legs and body
stop it from slipping backward.

Muscular back legs

OSTRICH LEG

An ostrich has the longest legs
and feet of any bird. A male's
legs may be up to 51 in (1.3 m)
long. Ostriches have only
two large toes on each foot,
and can run at speeds of up
to 43 mph (70 km/h).

Claw on larger toe

Toe bone

OX FRONT LEG

Oxen have thick, pillar-
like legs to support their
heavy bodies. Each leg
has only two toes (on the
rear legs) or fingers (on the
front legs). The lower limb
bones are fused for strength.
Each limb can support a
weight equivalent to three
adult humans.

Fingers tipped by two hooves (cloven hoof)

Dogfish swings its tail to propel itself through the water

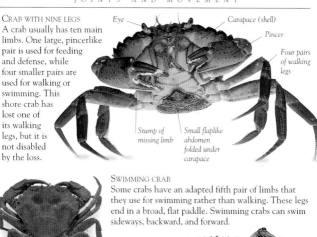

CRAB WITH NINE LEGS
A crab usually has ten main limbs. One large, pincerlike pair is used for feeding and defense, while four smaller pairs are used for walking or swimming. This shore crab has lost one of its walking legs, but it is not disabled by the loss.

Eye

Carapace (shell)

Pincer

Four pairs of walking legs

Stump of missing limb

Small flaplike abdomen folded under carapace

SWIMMING CRAB
Some crabs have an adapted fifth pair of limbs that they use for swimming rather than walking. These legs end in a broad, flat paddle. Swimming crabs can swim sideways, backward, and forward.

Swimming paddle

Tail processes provide attachment points for swimming muscles

ORCA
A killer whale, or orca, swims using its powerful tail. Orcas have no back legs, but many whales have a few leftover back leg bones, indicating that their ancestors once walked on land.

Flipper for steering and braking

SWIMMING SHARK
Sharks, such as this dogfish, swim by swinging their heads slightly and moving their tails from side to side. This creates an S-shaped wave that passes down the shark's body and pushes it through the water. The fish uses its pectoral fins to steer as it swims.

Pectoral fin

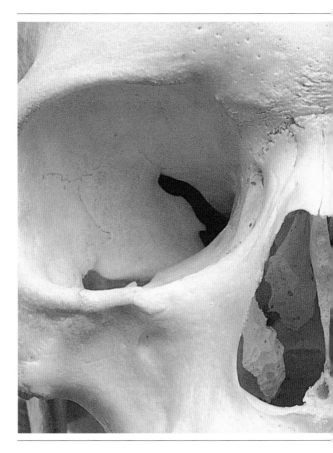

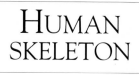

HUMAN SKELETON

PARTS OF THE SKELETON

THE HUMAN SKELETON, a framework of hard, interconnecting bones and softer cartilage, supports the body and protects its internal organs. It also provides an anchor for the muscles that enable the body to move. Each bone is a certain shape and size to suit the job that it has to do.

Frontal bone (forehead)

Orbit (eye socket)

Teeth

Nasal (nose) bone

Zygomatic (cheek) bone

Maxilla (upper jaw)

Mandible (lower jaw)

Clavicle (collarbone)

Sternum (breastbone)

Rib – attached to sternum

Costal cartilage

Three false ribs – attached to a true rib

Humerus (upper arm bone)

Floating rib

Radius (main forearm bone)

Ulna (lesser forearm bone)

Carpals (wrist bones)

Metacarpals (hand bones)

DEATH SYMBOL
Human skeletons are often used as symbols of death. This detail from a painting by Pieter Breughel (c. 1515–69) shows that not even the wealthy are immortal.

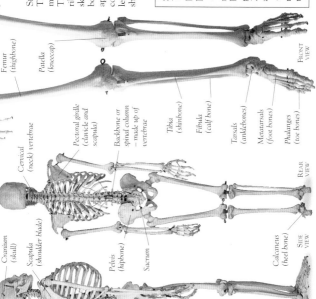

SKELETAL STRUCTURE

The skeleton has two main groups of bones. The skull, backbone, and ribcage form the axial skeleton, which is the body's upright axis. The appendicular skeleton consists of the arms and legs (appendages) and shoulder- and hipbones.

SKELETON FACTS

- Over half the body's bones are in the wrists, hands, ankles, and feet.

- A new baby has more than 300 bones but some fuse during growth to make about 206 bones in an adult skeleton.

- An adult's bones make up 14 percent of the body weight.

Phalanges (finger bones)

Femur (thighbone)

Patella (kneecap)

Pectoral girdle (clavicle and scapula)

Cervical (neck) vertebrae

Backbone or spinal column – made up of vertebrae

Tibia (shinbone)

Fibula (calf bone)

Tarsals (anklebones)

Metatarsals (foot bones)

Phalanges (toe bones)

FRONT VIEW

REAR VIEW

SIDE VIEW

Cranium (skull)

Scapula (shoulder blade)

Pelvis (hipbone)

Sacrum

Calcaneus (heel bone)

SKULL

THE SKULL is a hard casing of fused bones that surrounds and protects the brain and houses the sensory organs – the eyes, ears, and nose. It also provides openings for eating and breathing, as well as attachment points for the facial muscles and anchorage for the teeth.

Bones fully fused together at sutures

BABY'S SKULL
A baby's skull bones are not fully fused together, with soft areas (fontanelles) at the bone edges. This enables them to slide and overlap so the skull can change shape as the baby squeezes through the mother's pelvis during birth.

Sliding bones enable brain to grow rapidly

Fontanelles disappear at one year of age

BABY'S SKULL
FROM ABOVE

ADULT'S SKULL
FROM ABOVE

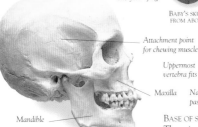

Attachment point for chewing muscle

Foramen magnum

Uppermost vertebra fits here

Maxilla *Nasal passages*

Mandible

SIDE VIEW OF SKULL
The upper jaw consists of two fixed bones that cannot move. The mandible is U-shaped and pivots on hinge joints just in front of the ears.

BASE OF SKULL
The spinal cord passes down from the brain through the spinal column through an oval hole at the base of the skull, the foramen magnum.

Roof of mouth

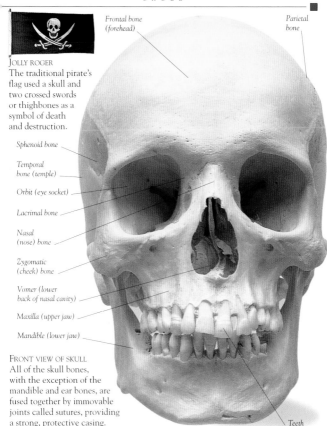

Frontal bone
(forehead)

Parietal
bone

JOLLY ROGER
The traditional pirate's
flag used a skull and
two crossed swords
or thighbones as a
symbol of death
and destruction.

Sphenoid bone

Temporal
bone (temple)

Orbit (eye socket)

Lacrimal bone

Nasal
(nose) bone

Zygomatic
(cheek) bone

Vomer (lower
back of nasal cavity)

Maxilla (upper jaw)

Mandible (lower jaw)

FRONT VIEW OF SKULL
All of the skull bones,
with the exception of the
mandible and ear bones,
are fused together by immovable
joints called sutures, providing
a strong, protective casing.

Teeth

4 3

Parts of the skull

The human skull is made up of 22 separate bones that fit tightly together like a jigsaw puzzle. There are eight bones in the cranium, or "brainbox," and 14 bones in the face. The maxilla consists of two bones on each side and the mandible has one bone on each side. Inside the skull are the ear bones, which are the smallest bones in the body.

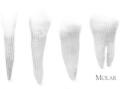

MOLAR

INCISOR   CANINE   PREMOLAR

TEETH

The full set of adult teeth totals 32, including incisors for cutting and slicing food, canines for gripping and tearing, and premolars and molars for crushing and chewing. Some people never develop the back four molars, or "wisdom teeth."

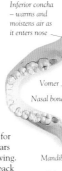

Inferior concha – warms and moistens air as it enters nose

Palatine – upper palate or back of roof of mouth

Vomer

Nasal bones

Mandible

Ethmoid bone – inner part of eye socket and back of nose

Maxilla

MALLEUS
(HAMMER)

INCUS
(ANVIL)

STAPES
(STIRRUP)

Malleus shown at actual size, on finger

EAR BONES

The three tiny bones, or ossicles, in the air-filled middle ear are often called by names that reflect their shape: hammer, anvil, and stirrup. The bones shake or vibrate when the eardrum vibrates, passing on these vibrations from the outer ear to the inner ear.

SKULL JIGSAW

The bones of the skull can be carefully separated to make it easier to see the many different bones. The zigzag edges of some bones show where they are locked together by sutures (see pp. 42–43). The lacrimal bone is not shown.

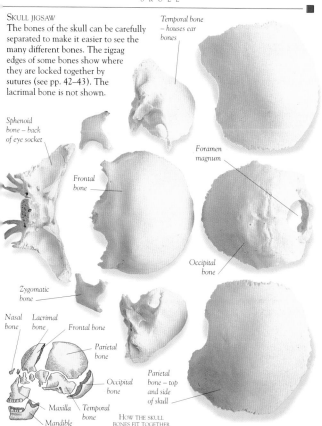

Temporal bone – houses ear bones

Sphenoid bone – back of eye socket

Foramen magnum

Frontal bone

Occipital bone

Zygomatic bone

Nasal bone *Lacrimal bone* *Frontal bone*

Parietal bone

Occipital bone

Maxilla *Temporal bone*

Mandible

Parietal bone – top and side of skull

HOW THE SKULL BONES FIT TOGETHER

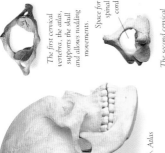

The first cervical vertebra, the atlas, supports the skull and allows nodding movements.

Space for spinal cord

The second cervical vertebra, the axis, allows side-to-side movement of the skull.

Vertebral arch

The other five cervical vertebrae are small and light. Their function is to support the head and neck.

Atlas

Axis

CERVICAL CURVE

SPINAL SHAPE
The spinal column is S-shaped with four main curves. These help to strengthen the backbone, balance the weight of the body, and absorb jolts during movement.

BACKBONE

THE HUMAN BACKBONE, or spinal column, consists of a row of 33 bones called vertebrae that surround and protect the spinal cord. The backbone also provides support for the head, arms, legs, and internal organs, and allows the upper body to bend, twist, and turn.

NECK STRETCHING
The Padaung people of Burma fit young girls with heavy brass neck rings to ward off evil spirits. The rings stretch the neck so much that it cannot support the head without them.

46

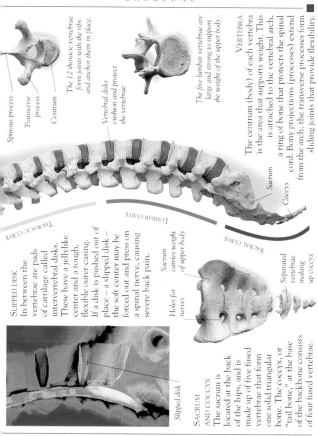

The 12 thoracic vertebrae form joints with the ribs and anchor them in place.

Spinous process

Transverse process

Centrum

The five lumbar vertebrae are large and strong to support the weight of the upper body.

Vertebral disks cushion and protect the vertebrae

VERTEBRA
The centrum (body) of each vertebra is the area that supports weight. This is attached to the vertebral arch, a ring of bone that protects the spinal cord. Bony projections (processes) extend from the arch; the transverse processes form sliding joints that provide flexibility.

THORACIC CURVE

LUMBAR CURVE

SACRAL CURVE

Sacrum

Coccyx

SLIPPED DISK
In between the vertebrae are pads of cartilage called intervertebral disks. These have a jellylike center and a tough, flexible outer casing. If a disk is pushed out of place – a slipped disk – the soft center may be forced out and press on a spinal nerve, causing severe back pain.

Sacrum carries weight of upper body

Holes for nerves

Separated vertebrae making up coccyx

Slipped disk

SACRUM AND COCCYX
The sacrum is located at the back of the hips, and is made up of five fused vertebrae that form one solid triangular bone. The coccyx, or "tail bone," at the base of the backbone consists of four fused vertebrae.

RIBS

THE RIBS are curved, flexible bones linked to form a protective cage around many of the internal organs. They also help the lungs to inflate and deflate during breathing. The 12 pairs of ribs are all attached to the backbone. Each rib is thin, flat, and springy to absorb shocks.

Socket in shoulder blade for upper arm bone

Scapula (shoulder blade

Rib 1

Head of rib

Neck of rib

RIB JOINTS
The ribs are joined to the backbone at flexible costovertebral joints. Each of these is a double joint. The neck of each rib fits into the transverse process of the vertebra, and the head of each rib fits into a socket on the centrum.

Ribs 1 to 7 are true ribs, joined to the breastbone by costal cartilage.

Ribs 8 to 10 are false ribs, joined to the ribs above.

Intervertebral disk

Centrum of vertebra

Socket

Transverse process of vertebra

Rib 7

SPARE RIB
According to the Old Testament, God created the first woman, Eve, from the spare rib of Adam, the first man.

Rib 8

Rib 10

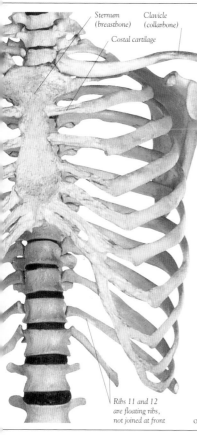

Sternum
(breastbone)

Clavicle
(collarbone)

Costal cartilage

Ribs 11 and 12
are floating ribs,
not joined at front

RIBBED FOR PROTECTION

The ribcage protects the
internal organs of the chest and
upper abdomen. The ribs are
closely spaced, with tough
ligaments and intercostal
muscles between them,
providing good protection
for the heart, lungs, liver,
and stomach.

Air is drawn in
down the windpipe

Left
lung

Intercostal muscles
contract, raising
ribs upward
and outward

Diaphragm
contracts
and flattens

BREATHING IN
(INHALATION)

Air is blown out
through the windpipe

Intercostal muscles
relax, moving ribs
inward and
downward

Diaphragm relaxes
into a dome

BREATHING OUT
(EXHALATION)

BREATHING MOTION

To breathe in, the intercostal
muscles and the diaphragm – a
muscle that forms the base of
the chest – contract. To breathe
out, the two sets of muscles relax.

SHOULDERS, ARMS, AND HANDS

THE BONES of the shoulders, arms, and hands have a wide range of functions. They enable people to pick up or throw objects, lift and carry heavy weights, play sports, make tools, or perform delicate, manipulative tasks, such as painting and drawing.

Scapula (shoulder blade)

Rounded head of humerus fits into socket in scapula to give all-around movement

Socket

ARM BONES
The bones of the arm are shaped according to the job they do. The wide, flat shoulder blade provides an area for muscle attachment, while the long arm bones can be extended to pick up objects. The many small hand bones allow delicate tasks to be performed.

Humerus

LEVER ACTION
The arm bones form a system of levers with pincers at the end. Holding a tennis racket makes the arm into an extra-long lever, and enables the tennis player to hit a ball with great force.

Elbow joint

RANGE OF MOVEMENT
The ball-and-socket joint in the shoulder enables the arm to move up and down, backward and forward, and around in a circle.

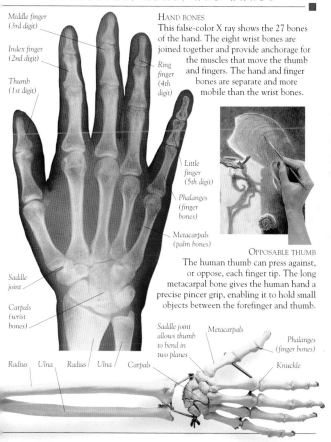

HAND BONES

This false-color X ray shows the 27 bones of the hand. The eight wrist bones are joined together and provide anchorage for the muscles that move the thumb and fingers. The hand and finger bones are separate and more mobile than the wrist bones.

Middle finger (3rd digit)

Index finger (2nd digit)

Thumb (1st digit)

Ring finger (4th digit)

Little finger (5th digit)

Phalanges (finger bones)

Metacarpals (palm bones)

Saddle joint

Carpals (wrist bones)

Radius   Ulna   Radius   Ulna   Carpals

OPPOSABLE THUMB

The human thumb can press against, or oppose, each finger tip. The long metacarpal bone gives the human hand a precise pincer grip, enabling it to hold small objects between the forefinger and thumb.

Saddle joint allows thumb to bend in two planes

Metacarpals

Phalanges (finger bones)

Knuckle

5 1

HIPS, LEGS, AND FEET

HUMAN LEG BONES must carry the body's weight, so they are bigger and stronger than the arm bones. At the top, they join onto the pelvis, which transmits the push of the legs to the upper body. The foot bones help keep the body balanced.

Head of femur

PELVIS

The pelvis is made up of the pelvic girdle, sacrum, and coccyx. Each side, or coxa, of the pelvic girdle consists of three fused bones – the ilium, ischium, and pubis. The human pelvis is unique, as it is rounded for walking upright.

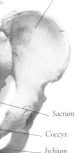

Base of spinal column

Ilium

Sacrum

Coccyx

Ischium

Socket for femur

Pubis

DOING THE SPLITS

Bones that meet at a joint are held in place by ligaments (see p. 32). Ballet dancers exercise to stretch their ligaments, enabling their thighbones to slide easily in and out of their hip joints.

LEFT COXA

Each coxa houses a deep socket for the head of the femur (thighbone). This gives great stability and strength to the hips, which bear all the weight of the upper body.

Socket for femur

Muscles attach here

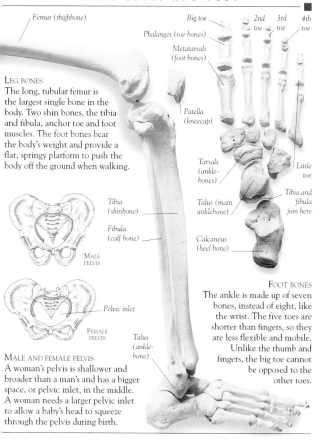

Femur (thighbone)

Big toe   2nd   3rd   4th
toe   toe   toe

Phalanges (toe bones)

Metatarsals (foot bones)

Patella (kneecap)

LEG BONES
The long, tubular femur is the largest single bone in the body. Two shin bones, the tibia and fibula, anchor toe and foot muscles. The foot bones bear the body's weight and provide a flat, springy platform to push the body off the ground when walking.

Tarsals (ankle-bones)

Little toe

Tibia (shinbone)

Fibula (calf bone)

Tibia and fibula join here

Talus (main anklebone)

Calcaneus (heel bone)

MALE PELVIS

FEMALE PELVIS

Pelvic inlet

Talus (ankle-bone)

FOOT BONES
The ankle is made up of seven bones, instead of eight, like the wrist. The five toes are shorter than fingers, so they are less flexible and mobile. Unlike the thumb and fingers, the big toe cannot be opposed to the other toes.

MALE AND FEMALE PELVIS
A woman's pelvis is shallower and broader than a man's and has a bigger space, or pelvic inlet, in the middle. A woman needs a larger pelvic inlet to allow a baby's head to squeeze through the pelvis during birth.

5 3

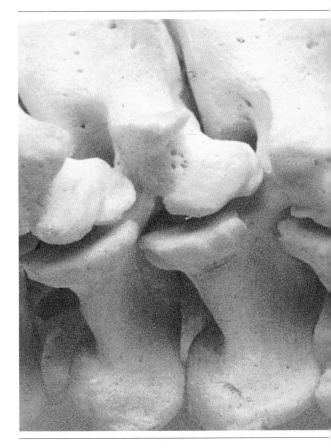

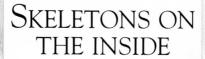

SKELETONS ON THE INSIDE

PRIMATES

WITH LARGE SKULLS to protect their big brains, members of the primate group, which includes humans, monkeys, gorillas, and lemurs, are arguably the most intelligent animals. Most primates live in the trees for some or all of the time and have long, strong finger and toe bones for gripping branches.

Incisor tooth

Wide eye sockets

Long middle finger

AYE-AYE
The nocturnal aye-aye has large eyes adapted for night vision, with wide, protective eye sockets. Its long middle finger and powerful incisor teeth enable it to dig out wood-boring insects from tree trunks.

Caudal (tail) vertebrae

Skull

Rounded cranium

Teeth adapted for eating fruit, seeds, and insects

NIGHT EYES
A loris's skull is dominated by its huge eye sockets, which are protected by a thick, bony ring called the orbital margin. Loris have a well-developed sense of smell to detect their slow-moving prey.

Orbital margin protects side of eye

DOUBLE LIFE
The rhesus macaque monkey spends time on the ground as well as in the trees. Its arm bones are as long as its leg bones, making walking easier. Tree-dwelling monkeys have longer back leg bones and a longer tail.

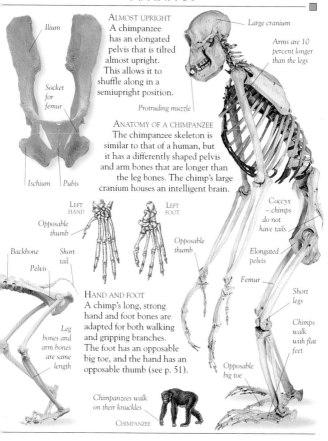

Ilium

Socket
for
femur

Ischium Pubis

ALMOST UPRIGHT
A chimpanzee
has an elongated
pelvis that is tilted
almost upright.
This allows it to
shuffle along in a
semiupright position.

Large cranium

Arms are 10
percent longer
than the legs

Protruding muzzle

ANATOMY OF A CHIMPANZEE
The chimpanzee skeleton is
similar to that of a human, but
it has a differently shaped pelvis
and arm bones that are longer than
the leg bones. The chimp's large
cranium houses an intelligent brain.

LEFT
HAND

LEFT
FOOT

Opposable
thumb

Coccyx
– chimps
do not
have tails

Elongated
pelvis

Femur

Short
legs

Chimps
walk
with flat
feet

Backbone
Pelvis

Short
tail

Opposable
thumb

Leg
bones and
arm bones
are same
length

HAND AND FOOT
A chimp's long, strong
hand and foot bones are
adapted for both walking
and gripping branches.
The foot has an opposable
big toe, and the hand has an
opposable thumb (see p. 51).

Opposable
big toe

Chimpanzees walk
on their knuckles

CHIMPANZEE

ELEPHANTS

THE SKELETON of an elephant has a strong backbone and pillarlike leg bones to support the animal's huge weight. Spinous processes form the shape of the back, which is concave in African elephants and convex in Asian elephants. The large skull supports the trunk and houses heavy, flat, grinding teeth.

Upper cranium

Rounded forehead

Molar teeth, with parallel ridges for grinding

Tusk sockets

Molar teeth

ELEPHANT'S JAW BONE
An elephant grinds up its food of coarse plants with four large molar teeth. As they wear out, new teeth slowly move forward from the back of the jaw to take their place. An elephant's teeth are replaced about six times in a lifetime.

ASIAN ELEPHANT LOWER JAW

Long spinous processes form convex back

Asian elephants have a concave forehead

Tusk

ASIAN ELEPHANT
The skeleton of this young Asian elephant has tusks, indicating it is a male. Female Asian elephants have much shorter tusks even when fully grown, or else they have no tusks at all.

ELEPHANT FACTS

• One tooth from an adult elephant is heavier than a brick, weighing about 10 lb (4.5 kg).

• Elephant tusks grow 7 in (17 cm) each year.

• Baby elephants lose their milk tusks when they are one year old.

MULTITUSK

This elephant skull, found in the Ituri forest in central Africa, has four tusks as a result of a rare deformity in the roots of the tusks. Elephants with up to seven tusks have been recorded.

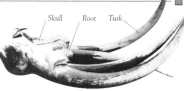

Skull Root Tusk

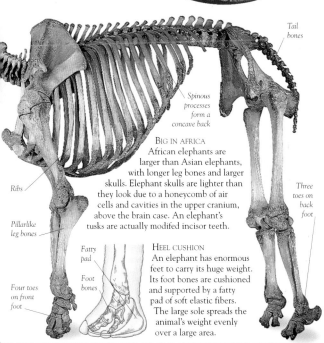

Tail bones

Spinous processes form a concave back

BIG IN AFRICA

African elephants are larger than Asian elephants, with longer leg bones and larger skulls. Elephant skulls are lighter than they look due to a honeycomb of air cells and cavities in the upper cranium, above the brain case. An elephant's tusks are actually modifed incisor teeth.

Ribs

Pillarlike leg bones

Three toes on back foot

Four toes on front foot

Fatty pad

Foot bones

HEEL CUSHION

An elephant has enormous feet to carry its huge weight. Its foot bones are cushioned and supported by a fatty pad of soft elastic fibers. The large sole spreads the animal's weight evenly over a large area.

HOOFED MAMMALS

INSTEAD OF CLAWS, all hoofed mammals, or ungulates, have hoofs of hard, protective horn. They also have fewer toes than other mammals. Ungulates balance on the tips of their toes and many, such as horses and antelopes, are fast runners, with long, thin leg bones.

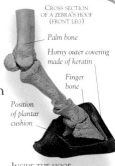

CROSS SECTION OF A ZEBRA'S HOOF (FRONT LEG)

Palm bone

Horny outer covering made of keratin

Finger bone

Position of plantar cushion

ODD-TOED MAMMALS

There are two main groups of hoofed mammals – odd-toed and even-toed. Odd-toed ungulates (perissodactyls), such as horses and rhinos, usually have either one or three toes (called "fingers" on the front legs) on each foot. The odd-toed tapir has three weight-bearing digits on its back feet and four on its front – the small fourth digit does not touch the ground.

Wrist bones

Wrist bones

Palm bones

Palm bone

Fourth digit

Finger bones

TAPIR FRONT LEG

Hoof

Single finger bone

SHETLAND PONY FRONT LEG

INSIDE THE HOOF

An ungulate's hoof surrounds and protects the animal's fragile toe or finger bones. A pad of fat (the plantar cushion) sandwiched between the hoof and bones acts as a shock absorber.

TWO-TOED MOVER

Even-toed ungulates (artiodactyls), such as oxen, gazelles, pigs, and camels, have two or four weight-bearing toes on each foot. This gazelle's ultrathin legs allow the animal to run at great speed.

Two finger bones

GAZELLE FRONT LEG

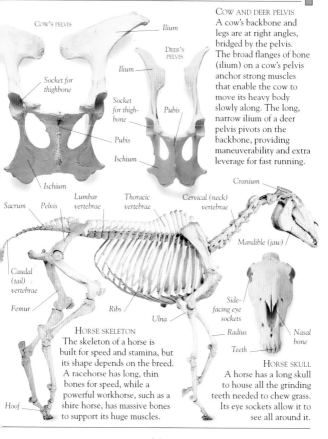

COW'S PELVIS

Ilium

DEER'S PELVIS

Ilium

Socket for thighbone

Socket for thighbone

Pubis

Pubis

Ischium

Ischium

COW AND DEER PELVIS

A cow's backbone and legs are at right angles, bridged by the pelvis. The broad flanges of bone (ilium) on a cow's pelvis anchor strong muscles that enable the cow to move its heavy body slowly along. The long, narrow ilium of a deer pelvis pivots on the backbone, providing maneuverability and extra leverage for fast running.

Cranium

Sacrum   Pelvis   Lumbar vertebrae   Thoracic vertebrae   Cervical (neck) vertebrae

Mandible (jaw)

Caudal (tail) vertebrae

Femur   Ribs   Ulna

Radius

Side-facing eye sockets

Nasal bone

Teeth

HORSE SKELETON

The skeleton of a horse is built for speed and stamina, but its shape depends on the breed. A racehorse has long, thin bones for speed, while a powerful workhorse, such as a shire horse, has massive bones to support its huge muscles.

Hoof

HORSE SKULL

A horse has a long skull to house all the grinding teeth needed to chew grass. Its eye sockets allow it to see all around it.

DOGS AND WOLVES

MEMBERS OF the dog family
(canids), which includes
wolves, dogs, and foxes, all
share similar skeletal features.
Canids have a large skull, a long
neck and backbone, and long leg
bones built for flexibility and
speed. Over the centuries, humans
have modified or exploited dog
anatomy through selective breeding.

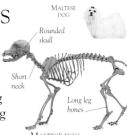

MALTESE
DOG

Rounded
skull

Short
neck

Long leg
bones

MALTESE DOG
All domesticated dogs
are descended from
wolves. This tiny Maltese
dog has a rounded skull
and shorter neck, but its
skeleton still resembles
that of a wolf.

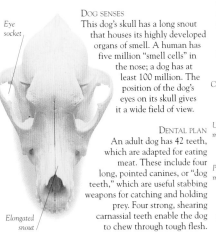

Eye
socket

Elongated
snout

DOG SENSES
This dog's skull has a long snout
that houses its highly developed
organs of smell. A human has
five million "smell cells" in
the nose; a dog has at
least 100 million. The
position of the dog's
eyes on its skull gives
it a wide field of view.

DENTAL PLAN
An adult dog has 42 teeth,
which are adapted for eating
meat. These include four
long, pointed canines, or "dog
teeth," which are useful stabbing
weapons for catching and holding
prey. Four strong, shearing
carnassial teeth enable the dog
to chew through tough flesh.

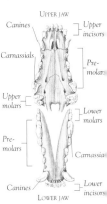

UPPER JAW

Canines

Upper
incisors

Carnassials

Premolars

Upper
molars

Lower
molars

Premolars

Carnassia

Canines

Lower
incisors

LOWER JAW

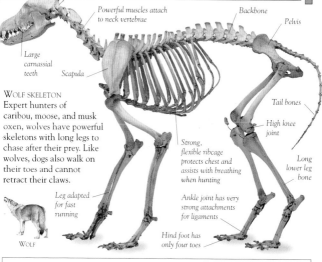

Powerful muscles attach
to neck vertebrae

Backbone

Pelvis

Large
carnassial
teeth

Scapula

Tail bones

High knee
joint

WOLF SKELETON
Expert hunters of
caribou, moose, and musk
oxen, wolves have powerful
skeletons with long legs to
chase after their prey. Like
wolves, dogs also walk on
their toes and cannot
retract their claws.

Strong,
flexible ribcage
protects chest and
assists with breathing
when hunting

Long
lower leg
bone

Leg adapted
for fast
running

Ankle joint has very
strong attachments
for ligaments

Hind foot has
only four toes

WOLF

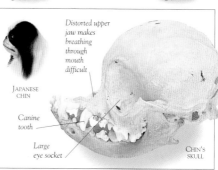

SELECTIVE BREEDING
Humans have bred
dogs with particular
features for centuries,
resulting in about 200
different breeds. Most
"toy dogs" are smaller
versions of larger
breeds in other groups.
Miniaturization
sometimes produces
strange skull shapes, as
in this Japanese Chin.

JAPANESE
CHIN

Distorted upper
jaw makes
breathing
through
mouth
difficult

Canine
tooth

Large
eye socket

CHIN'S
SKULL

CATS

ALTHOUGH THEY may vary in
size, all members of the cat family
are predators, with strong, supple
skeletons that are adapted for
hunting. Cats walk on their toes,
which enables them to move fast
when hunting. Powerful shoulders and
sharp claws help them grab hold of prey, which
they then kill with their long, pointed front teeth.

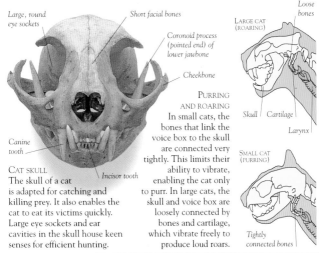

Long root of canine tooth

Cranium

Attachment for jaw muscles

Compressed neck vertebrae

Heavy lower jaw for powerful bite

Large, round eye sockets

Short facial bones

Coronoid process (pointed end) of lower jawbone

Cheekbone

Canine tooth

Incisor tooth

CAT SKULL
The skull of a cat
is adapted for catching and
killing prey. It also enables the
cat to eat its victims quickly.
Large eye sockets and ear
cavities in the skull house keen
senses for efficient hunting.

PURRING AND ROARING
In small cats, the
bones that link the
voice box to the skull
are connected very
tightly. This limits their
ability to vibrate,
enabling the cat only
to purr. In large cats, the
skull and voice box are
loosely connected by
bones and cartilage,
which vibrate freely to
produce loud roars.

Loose bones

LARGE CAT (ROARING)

Skull *Cartilage*

Larynx

SMALL CAT (PURRING)

Tightly connected bones

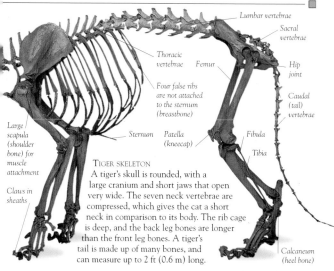

Lumbar vertebrae

Sacral vertebrae

Thoracic vertebrae

Femur

Hip joint

Four false ribs are not attached to the sternum (breastbone)

Caudal (tail) vertebrae

Large scapula (shoulder bone) for muscle attachment

Sternum

Patella (kneecap)

Fibula

Tibia

Claws in sheaths

Calcaneum (heel bone)

TIGER SKELETON
A tiger's skull is rounded, with a large cranium and short jaws that open very wide. The seven neck vertebrae are compressed, which gives the cat a short neck in comparison to its body. The rib cage is deep, and the back leg bones are longer than the front leg bones. A tiger's tail is made up of many bones, and can measure up to 2 ft (0.6 m) long.

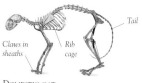

Tail

Claws in sheaths

Rib cage

DOMESTIC CAT
The skeleton of a domestic cat consists of about 250 bones. It is very similar to that of a tiger, although the rib cage is shallower. A small cat's tail is more flexible than a tiger's, and the sheaths around its claws are longer.

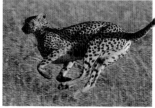

SPEEDY CAT
The cheetah, which can reach speeds of up to 60 mph (96 km/h), uses its long tail for balance and steering when running.

RODENTS AND RABBITS

MEMBERS OF the rodent group, including mice, squirrels, and guinea pigs, share a common feature with their close relatives, rabbits and hares – they all have continuously growing incisor teeth for gnawing. A typical rodent skeleton is a squat shape, with short legs and a long tail. Rabbit and hare skeletons have short tails and long back legs for leaping.

Strong, light skull

Curved cheek bones

Front teeth

Nasal passage

SQUIRREL
A tree squirrel has sharp claws for climbing and long back legs for leaping. The long tail helps with balance on tree branches and assists with steering when the squirrel leaps.

PACA SKULL
The paca is a nocturnal rodent from South America. It has curved, bowl-like cheek bones, the function of which is uncertain. It is thought they may amplify the sound that the paca makes. The honeycombed bone structure of the skull makes it strong but light.

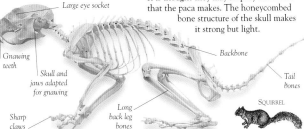

Large eye socket

Gnawing teeth

Skull and jaws adapted for gnawing

Backbone

Tail Bones

Sharp claws

Long back leg bones

SQUIRREL

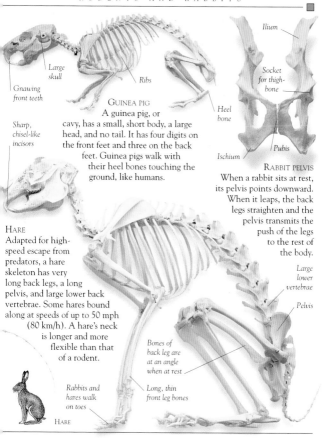

Large skull

Gnawing front teeth

Sharp, chisel-like incisors

Ribs

Heel bone

Ilium

Socket for thigh-bone

Ischium

Pubis

GUINEA PIG
A guinea pig, or cavy, has a small, short body, a large head, and no tail. It has four digits on the front feet and three on the back feet. Guinea pigs walk with their heel bones touching the ground, like humans.

RABBIT PELVIS
When a rabbit sits at rest, its pelvis points downward. When it leaps, the back legs straighten and the pelvis transmits the push of the legs to the rest of the body.

HARE
Adapted for high-speed escape from predators, a hare skeleton has very long back legs, a long pelvis, and large lower back vertebrae. Some hares bound along at speeds of up to 50 mph (80 km/h). A hare's neck is longer and more flexible than that of a rodent.

Large lower vertebrae

Pelvis

Bones of back leg are at an angle when at rest

Rabbits and hares walk on toes

Long, thin front leg bones

HARE

MARSUPIALS AND MONOTREMES

KANGAROOS and opossums are marsupials, mammals that rear their young in an external pouch attached to the abdominal wall. Marsupials have two epipubic bones on the pelvic girdle to support the abdominal wall. Monotremes, such as platypuses and anteaters, have epipubic bones, but their young hatch from eggs.

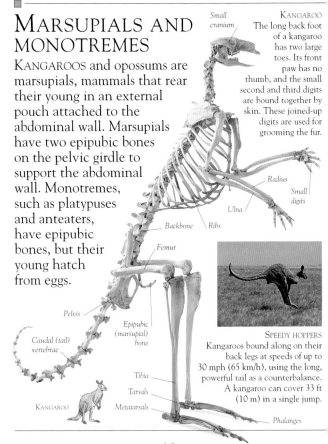

Small cranium

KANGAROO
The long back foot of a kangaroo has two large toes. Its front paw has no thumb, and the small second and third digits are bound together by skin. These joined-up digits are used for grooming the fur.

Radius

Small digits

Ulna

Backbone *Ribs*

Femur

Pelvis

Epipubic (marsupial) bone

Caudal (tail) vertebrae

Tibia

Tarsals

KANGAROO

Metatarsals

Phalanges

SPEEDY HOPPERS
Kangaroos bound along on their back legs at speeds of up to 30 mph (65 km/h), using the long, powerful tail as a counterbalance. A kangaroo can cover 33 ft (10 m) in a single jump.

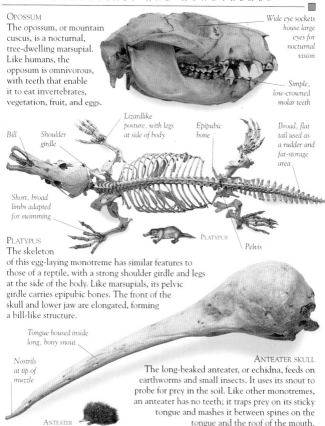

OPOSSUM
The opossum, or mountain cuscus, is a nocturnal, tree-dwelling marsupial. Like humans, the oppoosum is omnivorous, with teeth that enable it to eat invertebrates, vegetation, fruit, and eggs.

Wide eye sockets house large eyes for nocturnal vision

Simple, low-crowned molar teeth

Lizardlike posture, with legs at side of body

Epipubic bone

Broad, flat tail used as a rudder and fat-storage area

Bill

Shoulder girdle

Short, broad limbs adapted for swimming

PLATYPUS

Pelvis

PLATYPUS
The skeleton of this egg-laying monotreme has similar features to those of a reptile, with a strong shoulder girdle and legs at the side of the body. Like marsupials, its pelvic girdle carries epipubic bones. The front of the skull and lower jaw are elongated, forming a bill-like structure.

Tongue housed inside long, bony snout

Nostrils at tip of muzzle

ANTEATER

ANTEATER SKULL
The long-beaked anteater, or echidna, feeds on earthworms and small insects. It uses its snout to probe for prey in the soil. Like other monotremes, an anteater has no teeth; it traps prey on its sticky tongue and mashes it between spines on the tongue and the roof of the mouth.

SEA MAMMALS

FROM SEALS and walruses to whales and dolphins, sea mammal skeletons are adapted to an aquatic lifestyle. Their limbs have evolved into flippers, with long finger and toe bones. Whales and dolphins are supported by water, so their skeletons are used mainly to anchor muscles.

Thoracic vertebrae

BIG TOOTH
An adult male sperm whale has the largest teeth of any animal. A tooth can grow to 10 in (25 cm) long. There are usually 35–50 teeth in total.

A true seal swims using back flippers

Lumbar vertebrae

SEAL
A true seal has large lumbar vertebrae to anchor the muscles of its propelling back flippers. Fur seals and sea lions swim with their front flippers and have large cervical and thoracic vertebrae for anchorage.

Small front flippers used for steering

PYGMY RIGHT WHALE
A whale skeleton has a long skull, short neck, and no back legs. The dorsal fin and the powerful tail flukes do not contain bones. Whale bones are light and spongy as they do not have to support the weight of the animal.

PYGMY RIGHT WHALE

Vestigial leg bone – remains of back legs

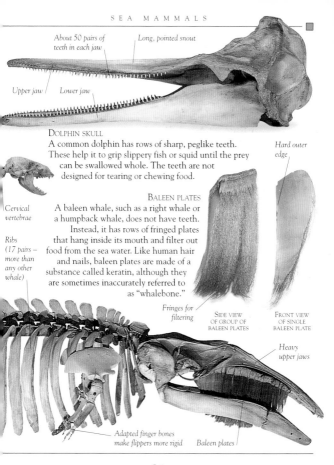

About 50 pairs of
teeth in each jaw

Long, pointed snout

Upper jaw

Lower jaw

DOLPHIN SKULL
A common dolphin has rows of sharp, peglike teeth.
These help it to grip slippery fish or squid until the prey
can be swallowed whole. The teeth are not
designed for tearing or chewing food.

Hard outer
edge

Cervical
vertebrae

BALEEN PLATES
A baleen whale, such as a right whale or
a humpback whale, does not have teeth.
Instead, it has rows of fringed plates
that hang inside its mouth and filter out
food from the sea water. Like human hair
and nails, baleen plates are made of a
substance called keratin, although they
are sometimes inaccurately referred to
as "whalebone."

Ribs
(17 pairs –
more than
any other
whale)

Fringes for
filtering

SIDE VIEW
OF GROUP OF
BALEEN PLATES

FRONT VIEW
OF SINGLE
BALEEN PLATE

Heavy
upper jaws

Adapted finger bones
make flippers more rigid

Baleen plates

BIRDS

MOST BIRD SKELETONS are adapted
for flight. The arm bones form wings,
and a large, keel-like breastbone
provides anchorage for the
powerful flight muscles. Bird
skeletons are lightweight, with
many fused bones that form
a rigid frame. A horny beak
takes the place of a heavy
jawbone and teeth.

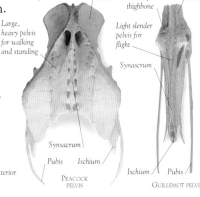

Large eye socket

Cranium

Cervical vertebrae

Lightweight beak

Ilium   Socket for thighbone   Ilium

Light slender pelvis for flight

Synsacrum

Large, heavy pelvis for walking and standing

Synsacrum

Pubis   Ischium

PEACOCK PELVIS

Ischium / Pubis

GUILLEMOT PELVIS

SKULL BONE   Dense interior

Air-filled space

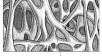

WING BONE   Lightweight interior

BONE STRUCTURE

A bird's pelvis, wing bones, and parts
of the skull are hollow. Although they
vary in density, they are all formed
from a honeycombed network of air
spaces and supporting struts.

ADAPTED PELVIS

In all birds, the pelvic bones are fused
to the lower vertebrae, forming the
synsacrum. The shape of the pelvis varies
between species according to its function.

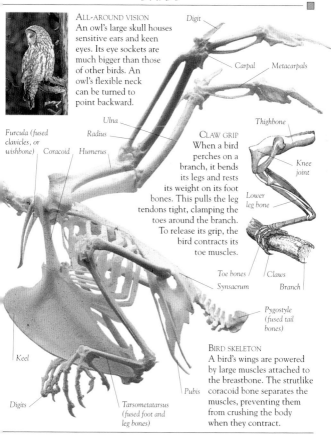

ALL-AROUND VISION
An owl's large skull houses sensitive ears and keen eyes. Its eye sockets are much bigger than those of other birds. An owl's flexible neck can be turned to point backward.

Digit

Carpal Metacarpals

Ulna

Radius

Thighbone

Furcula (fused clavicles, or wishbone)

Coracoid Humerus

Knee joint

Lower leg bone

CLAW GRIP
When a bird perches on a branch, it bends its legs and rests its weight on its foot bones. This pulls the leg tendons tight, clamping the toes around the branch. To release its grip, the bird contracts its toe muscles.

Toe bones Claws

Synsacrum Branch

Pygostyle (fused tail bones)

Keel

Pubis

Digits

Tarsometatarsus (fused foot and leg bones)

BIRD SKELETON
A bird's wings are powered by large muscles attached to the breastbone. The strutlike coracoid bone separates the muscles, preventing them from crushing the body when they contract.

REPTILES

MOST REPTILES, such as lizards, crocodiles, and chameleons, have a long, lizardlike skeleton, with a flexible backbone and short legs that stick out sideways. There are, however, exceptions. Snakes have no limbs, and turtles and tortoises have an external shell as well as an internal skeleton.

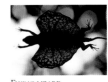

FLYING LIZARD
This flying dragon lizard (*Draco volans*) glides from tree to tree to escape its enemies. Its "wings" are made of skin and are strengthened by five ribs on each side.

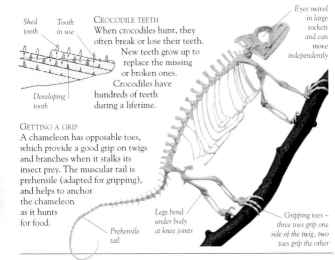

Shed tooth

Tooth in use

Developing tooth

CROCODILE TEETH
When crocodiles hunt, they often break or lose their teeth. New teeth grow up to replace the missing or broken ones. Crocodiles have hundreds of teeth during a lifetime.

GETTING A GRIP
A chameleon has opposable toes, which provide a good grip on twigs and branches when it stalks its insect prey. The muscular tail is prehensile (adapted for gripping), and helps to anchor the chameleon as it hunts for food.

Eyes swivel in large sockets and can move independently

Legs bend under body at knee joints

Prehensile tail

Gripping toes – three toes grip one side of the twig, two toes grip the other

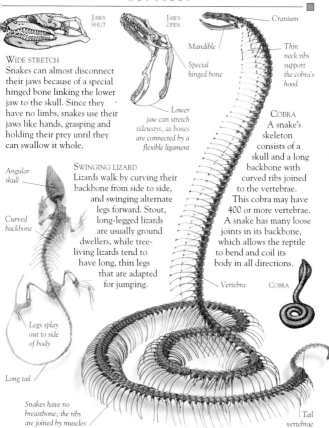

JAWS SHUT

JAWS OPEN

Cranium

Mandible

Special hinged bone

Thin neck ribs support the cobra's hood

WIDE STRETCH

Snakes can almost disconnect their jaws because of a special hinged bone linking the lower jaw to the skull. Since they have no limbs, snakes use their jaws like hands, grasping and holding their prey until they can swallow it whole.

Lower jaw can stretch sideways, as bones are connected by a flexible ligament

COBRA

A snake's skeleton consists of a skull and a long backbone with curved ribs joined to the vertebrae. This cobra may have 400 or more vertebrae. A snake has many loose joints in its backbone, which allows the reptile to bend and coil its body in all directions.

Angular skull

Curved backbone

SWINGING LIZARD

Lizards walk by curving their backbone from side to side, and swinging alternate legs forward. Stout, long-legged lizards are usually ground dwellers, while tree-living lizards tend to have long, thin legs that are adapted for jumping.

Legs splay out to side of body

Long tail

Snakes have no breastbone; the ribs are joined by muscles

Vertebra

COBRA

Tail vertebrae

AMPHIBIANS

THE SKELETONS OF most amphibian species fall into three main categories. These include salamander-type, with a broad skull, long body and tail, and short legs; frog-type; with a broad skull, short body, no tail, and long back legs; and caecilian-type, which has a narrow skull, long backbone, and no legs.

Orbit (eye socket)

Short backbone

Long foot bones

Urostyle

Elongated anklebone

JUMPING FROG
A frog skeleton is adapted for jumping and swimming. It has long leg, feet, and toe bones, including two elongated anklebones that allow the back legs to bend for jumping. The broad skull has large eye sockets, and the tail vertebrae are fused to form a rodlike bone called the urostyle.

Top row of front teeth

SKULL OF A SIREN
Sirens are eel-like amphibians with small front legs but no back legs. Unlike frogs and salamanders, their lower jaw teeth are on an inner bone. They do not have an bony arch around their eye sockets, and their jaws are covered with a horny outer coating.

Palate, or roof of mouth

Eye socket

Lower jaw teeth on inner bone

SIREN'S SKULL WITH MOUTH CLOSED

SIREN'S SKULL WITH MOUTH OPEN

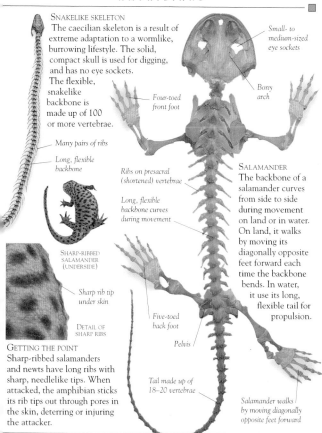

SNAKELIKE SKELETON
The caecilian skeleton is a result of extreme adaptation to a wormlike, burrowing lifestyle. The solid, compact skull is used for digging, and has no eye sockets. The flexible, snakelike backbone is made up of 100 or more vertebrae.

Small- to medium-sized eye sockets

Bony arch

Four-toed front foot

Many pairs of ribs

Long, flexible backbone

Ribs on presacral (shortened) vertebrae

Long, flexible backbone curves during movement

SHARP-RIBBED SALAMANDER (UNDERSIDE)

Sharp rib tip under skin

DETAIL OF SHARP RIBS

SALAMANDER
The backbone of a salamander curves from side to side during movement on land or in water. On land, it walks by moving its diagonally opposite feet forward each time the backbone bends. In water, it use its long, flexible tail for propulsion.

Five-toed back foot

Pelvis

GETTING THE POINT
Sharp-ribbed salamanders and newts have long ribs with sharp, needlelike tips. When attacked, the amphibian sticks its rib tips out through pores in the skin, deterring or injuring the attacker.

Tail made up of 18–20 vertebrae

Salamander walks by moving diagonally opposite feet forward

BONY FISH

MOST FISH, such as cod, carp, and
salmon, have an internal skeleton
made of bone. Strong muscles
attached to a flexible backbone
bend the body from side to side to
push the fish along. Fish do not have
limb bones; instead, they use their
movable fins and flexible tail to swim
through the water.

Fin rays

Vertebra

Ribs

SKELETON
OF LEMON SOLE

RAZOR TEETH
Piranhas have triangular,
razor-sharp teeth to carve
slices of flesh from their
prey. When a piranha
closes its jaws, its teeth
snap together in a strong
bite. Most piranhas
eat meat only
when plant
food is scarce.

*Lower jaw teeth are larger
than upper jaw teeth*

*Caudal
(tail) fin*

*Fins are made up of
many skeletal rays*

EEL SKELETON
A conger eel's flexible backbone is made
up of 100 or more vertebrae. Its skeleton
has no pelvic or tail fins, and many
species have no pectoral fins either.
The dorsal and anal fins
form a continuous
fringe around
the body.

CONGER EEL

Sharp teeth

*Great numbers of
vertebrae in backbone
for flexibility*

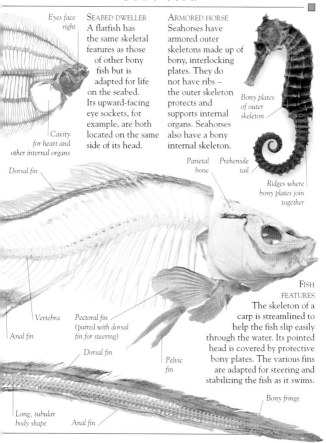

Eyes face right

Cavity for heart and other internal organs

SEABED DWELLER
A flatfish has the same skeletal features as those of other bony fish but is adapted for life on the seabed. Its upward-facing eye sockets, for example, are both located on the same side of its head.

ARMORED HORSE
Seahorses have armored outer skeletons made up of bony, interlocking plates. They do not have ribs – the outer skeleton protects and supports internal organs. Seahorses also have a bony internal skeleton.

Bony plates of outer skeleton

Prehensile tail

Parietal bone

Ridges where bony plates join together

Dorsal fin

Vertebra

Pectoral fin (paired with dorsal fin for steering)

Anal fin

Dorsal fin

Pelvic fin

FISH FEATURES
The skeleton of a carp is streamlined to help the fish slip easily through the water. Its pointed head is covered by protective bony plates. The various fins are adapted for steering and stabilizing the fish as it swims.

Bony fringe

Long, tubular body shape

Anal fin

SHARKS AND RAYS

THE SKELETONS of about 700 fish species, including sharks, skates, and rays, are made of strong, flexible cartilage (gristle) instead of bone. Cartilaginous fish have hinged jaws, but the teeth are not fused to the jaws. Their vertebrae are formed by layers of cartilage around the spinal cord. They are nearly all predators that live in salt water.

Centrum

Network of fibers

BASKER'S BACKBONE
This is the centrum of a vertebra from a basking shark, strengthened by a network of mineral-laced fibers. The basking shark is the second largest fish in the world, reaching up to 45 ft (15 m) in length.

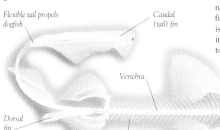

Flexible tail propels dogfish

Caudal (tail) fin

Vertebra

Cranium

Dorsal fin

Rib

Pectoral fin

DOGFISH
The cartilaginous skeleton of a dogfish is similar to that of a bony fish, but less rigid. The flexible tail is adapted for fast swimming, bending from side to side to speed the fish through the water.

RAY SKELETON
Like sharks, rays have a cartilaginous skeleton. Flexible, skeletal "rays" form winglike pectoral fins, which the fish uses for propulsion.

Framework of "rays"

Pectoral fin

Tail

SHARK'S TEETH

Predatory sharks, such as the great white, have large, razor-sharp, serrated teeth. Other sharks have flat teeth to crush shells or long, thin teeth to hold slippery fish. Sharks' teeth grow continuously – a shark may use over 20,000 teeth in its lifetime.

Teeth ready for use

Old teeth wear out

TEETH OF MAKO SHARK

Teeth developing within jaw

GREAT WHITE SHARK JAWS

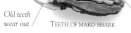

Placoid scales (small "teeth") made from modified denticles

Placoid scales are found along the gills and in the throat and gullet

TINY TEETH

The whale shark is the world's biggest fish, but it has some of the smallest "teeth." These modified denticles (skin scales) are called placoid scales, and are used to sieve small, floating creatures from the water.

Cutaway of snout shows sharp saw teeth in cartilage sockets

Sawfish snout

SAW TEETH

A sawfish has 12 to 30 pairs of razor-sharp teeth growing on its snout, as well as flat, crushing teeth in its jaws. Sawfish use their snout both to capture food and as a defensive weapon.

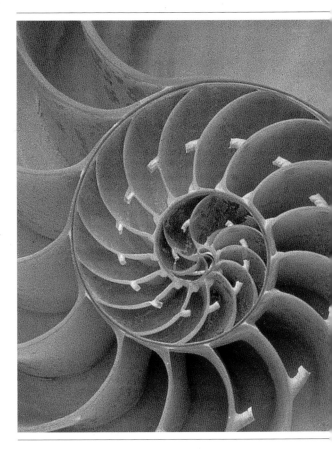

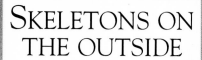

SKELETONS ON THE OUTSIDE

ECHINODERMS AND MOLLUSKS

ECHINODERMS, such as starfish and sea urchins, have spiny bodies and a skeleton made of hard plates, called ossicles, underneath the skin. The ossicles may be movable or fused together. Soft-bodied mollusks, such as snails and cockles, have a protective external skeleton, called a shell. Mollusk shells are made from calcium carbonate.

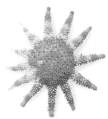

SUNSTAR
The skeleton of a starfish, such as this sunstar, is made up of separate ossicles that are shaped like rods, crosses, or plates. The ossicles are arranged in a lattice network and are joined together by connective tissue.

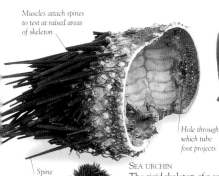

Muscles attach spines to test at raised areas of skeleton

Hole through which tube foot projects

Spine

CALIFORNIAN PURPLE SEA URCHIN

Test with spines removed

SEA URCHIN
The rigid skeleton of a sea urchin, called a test, is made up of many interlocking crystals. In living sea urchins, the outside of the test is covered with spines for protection and tube feet for movement.

BIVALVE MOLLUSK

The shell of a bivalve is divided into two parts, called valves. In this common cockle, the valves are connected by ridged teeth that form a hinge. Strong muscles and ligaments open and close the valves. Thick ribs help to strengthen the outer structure of the shell.

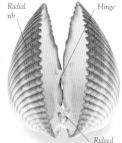

Radial rib

Hinge

Ridged teeth

MOLLUSK FACTS

• The largest land snail is the African giant snail, with a shell that grows up to 8 in (20 cm) long.

• Most land snails eat plants, but the *Euglandina* snail uses its long, sharp teeth to eat other snails.

A snail's soft internal organs are protected by its shell

LAND SNAIL

Land snails usually have thinner, lighter shells than their shelled relatives in the sea, as they are not supported by water. A land snail can retreat inside its shell to escape danger or to survive cold or dry weather.

Most snail shells are coiled into a spiral shape

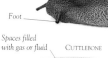
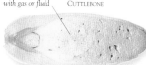

Tentacle

Eye

Head

Foot

Spaces filled with gas or fluid

CUTTLEBONE

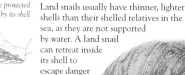

CUTTLEFISH

A cuttlefish "bone" is in fact the animal's internal shell. The cuttlefish controls its movement by filling the many spaces in the shell with gas to make it rise, or fluid to make it sink.

CUTTLEFISH

CRUSTACEANS

CRABS, SHRIMPS, lobsters,
barnacles, and wood lice are all
crustaceans. Their tough, external
skeleton, or exoskeleton, is
covered with a hard outer "crust"
made from chitin strengthened
with calcium carbonate. Most
crustaceans have sections of thin,
flexible skin at the leg joints to
allow movement.

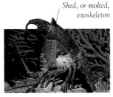

*Shed, or molted,
exoskeleton*

MOLTING
Crustaceans grow by forming
a new, bigger exoskeleton
under the old one. To molt
the exoskeleton, the animal
takes in water to swell its
body. This causes the new
skeleton to burst through
the old one.

Soft abdomen

*Hermit crab in
transparent shell*

*Hook on tip of
abdomen grips
inside of shell*

*Pointed
feet*

Small claw

Carapace

*Large
pincer
claw*

HERMIT CRAB
Unlike most crabs, the hermit
crab does not have a hard outer
shell on its abdomen. This makes it
vulnerable, and so it lives inside empty
mollusk shells for extra protection. As it
grows larger, the crab may change its
cramped shell for a bigger one.

*Large
pincer
blocks
entrance
to shell*

MUSICAL CRAB
The fiddler crab
has an oversized claw
that it uses to warn off rival
males or attract females.
The smaller claw is used for
feeding. Like other crabs,
it has a wide, hard shield
called a carapace to protect
the front of its body.

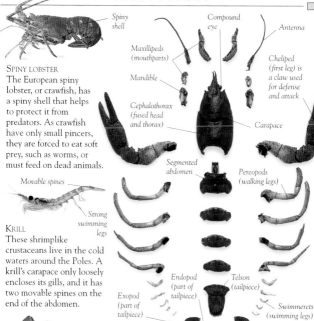

Spiny shell

Compound eye

Antenna

Maxillipeds (mouthparts)

Mandible

Cheliped (first leg) is a claw used for defense and attack

Cephalothorax (fused head and thorax)

Carapace

Segmented abdomen

Pereopods (walking legs)

Endopod (part of tailpiece)

Telson (tailpiece)

Exopod (part of tailpiece)

Swimmerets (swimming legs)

SPINY LOBSTER

The European spiny lobster, or crawfish, has a spiny shell that helps to protect it from predators. As crawfish have only small pincers, they are forced to eat soft prey, such as worms, or must feed on dead animals.

Movable spines

Strong swimming legs

KRILL

These shrimplike crustaceans live in the cold waters around the Poles. A krill's carapace only loosely encloses its gills, and it has two movable spines on the end of the abdomen.

Plates thicken and widen as barnacle grows

BARNACLES

To protect their bodies and limbs, most barnacles have a set of shell-like plates that can be opened or closed. The barnacle's legs can be pushed outside to catch food or drawn back inside for protection.

CRAYFISH

Most crustaceans, such as this crayfish, have a segmented body with hard, overlapping plates that form an armored exoskeleton. The large carapace plate protects both the head and the thorax (middle part of the body).

INSECTS

THERE ARE many types of insect exoskeletons, ranging from the hard outer case of a beetle to the soft, stretchy skin of a caterpillar. Made of waterproof chitin, the strong, protective exoskeleton supports the insect and has flexible joints that allow a wide range of movement. It cannot expand – the insect molts its exoskeleton in order to grow.

Soft new exoskeleton

Blood is pumped into the thorax to make it swell

Old exoskeleton

MOLTING
To shed its skin, a caterpillar takes in air or water to expand its body. This splits the old exoskeleton, which the insect then wriggles free of, using its muscles.

Leg muscles are inside leg skeleton

MOLTING SEQUENCE
When a damselfly hatches out of its egg, it resembles a tiny adult. Called a nymph, it lives underwater and molts its skin several times as it grows. The final molt into an adult takes place out of water.

Elytra (hard wing cases)

Thorax

Wing-bud case

Plant stem

GOLIATH BEETLE
Exoskeletons are a major reason for the small size of insects. The Goliath beetle is the heaviest insect, but it is still fairly small. If the exoskeleton were any larger, it would be too thick and heavy for the insect's muscles to move.

Abdomen

HOLDING ON
The nymph clings to a plant stem above the water. The wings are folded inside the wing-bud case.

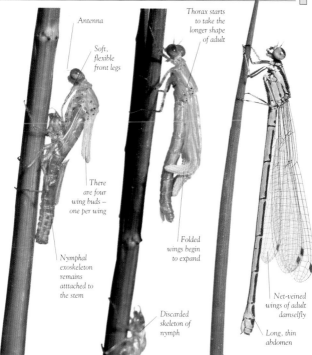

Antenna

Soft, flexible front legs

Thorax starts to take the longer shape of adult

There are four wing buds – one per wing

Nymphal exoskeleton remains atttached to the stem

Folded wings begin to expand

Discarded skeleton of nymph

Net-veined wings of adult damselfly

Long, thin abdomen

BREAKING FREE
Most of the top part of the body has pulled free of the nymphal exoskeleton, which remains attached to the stem.

GROWING UP
Blood is pumped into the wings to make them expand and grow longer. The thorax is also longer, more like the adult shape.

FULLY FLEDGED
About two hours after the nymph first crawls out of the water, it is ready to fly. Its bright colors develop after a few days.

Types of insects

There are at least five million different types, or species, of insects. They all have six jointed legs, and most of them have two pairs of wings. Insect exoskeletons have plated body segments and tubular legs. The size, shape, and color of an insect's exoskeleton varies between species to suit their different methods of movement, feeding, defense, and mate attraction.

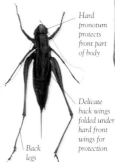

Hard pronotum protects front part of body

STICK INSECT

Delicate back wings folded under hard front wings for protection

Back legs

JUMPING GRASSHOPPER
The long, powerful back legs of a grasshopper enable it to leap away from danger. If it is caught by one of its back legs, it can break off the leg to escape. The wound in the exoskeleton seals immediately.

INSECT CAMOUFLAGE
The long, slender, green or brown exoskeleton of a stick insect helps it to blend into a background of leaves and twigs. Predators find it hard to see through this disguise. Leaf insects are related to stick insects, but have flat bodies and leaflike leg flaps.

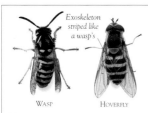

Exoskeleton striped like a wasp's

WASP   HOVERFLY

MIMICRY
Some harmless insects protect themselves by mimicking the appearance of dangerous ones. A hoverfly's exoskeleton resembles that of a poisonous wasp. Predators mistake the harmless hoverfly for the dangerous wasp and leave it alone.

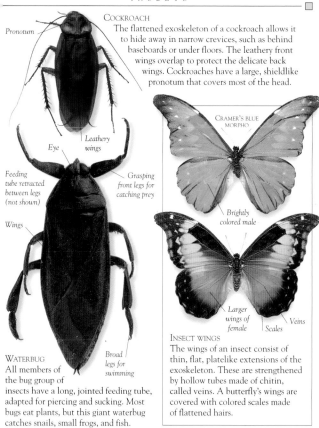

COCKROACH

The flattened exoskeleton of a cockroach allows it to hide away in narrow crevices, such as behind baseboards or under floors. The leathery front wings overlap to protect the delicate back wings. Cockroaches have a large, shieldlike pronotum that covers most of the head.

Pronotum

Eye

Leathery wings

CRAMER'S BLUE MORPHO

Brightly colored male

Feeding tube retracted between legs (not shown)

Grasping front legs for catching prey

Wings

Larger wings of female

Scales

Veins

WATERBUG

All members of the bug group of insects have a long, jointed feeding tube, adapted for piercing and sucking. Most bugs eat plants, but this giant waterbug catches snails, small frogs, and fish.

Broad legs for swimming

INSECT WINGS

The wings of an insect consist of thin, flat, platelike extensions of the exoskeleton. These are strengthened by hollow tubes made of chitin, called veins. A butterfly's wings are covered with colored scales made of flattened hairs.

ARACHNIDS

LIKE INSECTS, arachnids
molt their exoskeletons
in order to grow. All
arachnids have four pairs
of jointed walking legs
and an exoskeleton divided
into two body sections.
Instead of jaws, they have
chelicerae (pincerlike
mouthparts) and pedipalps
(frontal appendages).

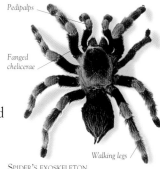

Pedipalps

Fanged
chelicerae

Walking legs

SPIDER'S EXOSKELETON
Unlike other arachnids, a spider's
chelicerae have powerful fangs, which it
uses to inject deadly venom into its prey.

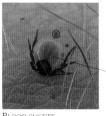

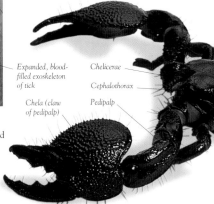

BLOOD SUCKER
A tick is a tiny arachnid
that feeds by sucking blood
from animals. Its highly
folded exoskeleton can
expand greatly during
feeding, allowing the
tick to consume as much
blood as possible.

Expanded, blood-
filled exoskeleton
of tick

Chela (claw
of pedipalp)

Chelicerae

Cephalothorax

Pedipalp

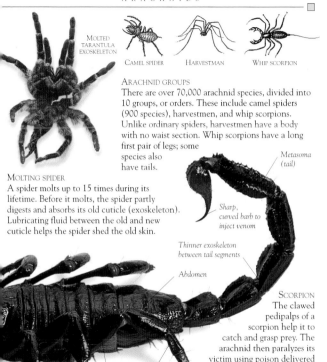

MOLTED
TARANTULA
EXOSKELETON

CAMEL SPIDER   HARVESTMAN   WHIP SCORPION

ARACHNID GROUPS

There are over 70,000 arachnid species, divided into 10 groups, or orders. These include camel spiders (900 species), harvestmen, and whip scorpions. Unlike ordinary spiders, harvestmen have a body with no waist section. Whip scorpions have a long first pair of legs; some species also have tails.

Metasoma
(tail)

Sharp,
curved barb to
inject venom

MOLTING SPIDER

A spider molts up to 15 times during its lifetime. Before it molts, the spider partly digests and absorbs its old cuticle (exoskeleton). Lubricating fluid between the old and new cuticle helps the spider shed the old skin.

Thinner exoskeleton
between tail segments

Abdomen

SCORPION

The clawed pedipalps of a scorpion help it to catch and grasp prey. The arachnid then paralyzes its victim using poison delivered by a stinger on the end of its tail. Thinner sections of exoskeleton between the tail segments enable the tail to bend forward to sting the prey.

Tibia

Femur

Patella   Metatarsus

Tarsus

Walking leg

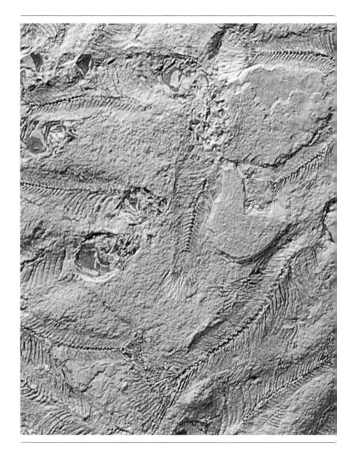

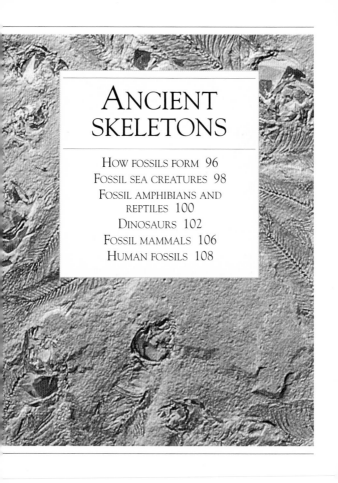

ANCIENT SKELETONS

HOW FOSSILS FORM

FOSSILS ARE the preserved
evidence of once-living
animals or plants. The
most common fossils are
hard skeletal remains,
such as bones, teeth, or shells.
The soft tissues of an organism
rot away and are rarely preserved.
The word *fossil* means "dug out of
the ground," as most fossils
are discovered within
layers of rock.

SPIDER IN AMBER
Amber is a sticky
tree resin that
sometimes traps
small creatures and
preserves them as it
hardens. This fossil
spider was trapped in amber
20–30 million years ago.

*Bony,
protective
neck frill* *Eye
socket* *Bony
horn*

*Row of
slicing teeth*

A Triceratops
dies and its bones
are picked clean
by meat-eaters.

*The skull is
buried in the mud and sand
of the riverbed. The rest of
the skeleton is destroyed.*

TRICERATOPS
Many extinct
species are preserved as
fossils. This fossil skull is of a
plant-eating dinosaur called *Triceratops*,
which died out 65 million years ago. Its
fossilized skeletal remains give us clues
as to what it looked like and how it lived.

FOSSILIZATION ON LAND
The remains of land animals
usually decay, are eaten by scavengers,
or are scattered by wind and water,
making fossils rare. Most fossils of land
animals are found either in sediments at
the bottom of lakes or rivers, in natural
tar pits, or in frozen soil.

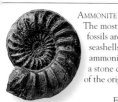

AMMONITE

The most common fossils are ancient seashells. This ammonite fossil is a stone cast of the outside of the original shell.

Shell fragments may not fossilize

Living ammonite

After death, shell sinks

FOSSILIZATION AT SEA

Fossils are often formed on the sea floor. Dead plants and animals are buried under layers of sand, mud, and other sediment, which preserve the remains. As the layers of soft sediment turn into hard sedimentary rock, the remains also usually turn to stone.

Shell chemically altered

Shell dissolves and cast is formed

Buried shell preserved intact

Earth movements 15,000 years ago have pushed the fossil skull closer to the surface. An ice age occurs.

Woolly mammoth

After 15 million years, the buried skull has turned into a hard, stony fossil. On the land above, mammals have taken over from dinosaurs.

Today, wind and rain have worn away the rocks above the fossil skull. Fossil hunters now begin to dig the skull out of the rock.

FOSSIL SEA CREATURES

SOME OF THE most common fossils are
the skeletons of fish and animals without
backbones (invertebrates). Fossilized
remains include ancient sea creatures that
died out millions of years ago, as well
as species that are still alive today.

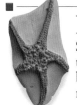

STARFISH
This *Stauranderaster*
fossil is rare in that it
has been preserved
intact; the hard plates
(ossicles) that make
up its body are usually
scattered after death.

TRILOBITES
These marine arthropods
had a hard, distinctive
external skeleton. Like
modern crustaceans, insects,
and arachnids, trilobites had
to molt in order to grow.
Many fossils are pieces of
molted skeleton. Trilobites
died out about 245 million
years ago.

*Segmented body
rolled up for safety*

*Large
compound
eye*

*A trilobite – meaning
"three lobes" – had a
body divided
into three
parts.*

Head

*Tail locking
into groove
under head
for protection*

Eye

Bony head shield

UNROLLED
TRILOBITE

FISH WITHOUT JAWS
Jawless fish were the first
animals with backbones
(vertebrates). They lived
400 million years ago, and fed by
sucking up food from the sea bed.
Many of them, like this *Cephalaspis*,
had bony scales and a head shield.

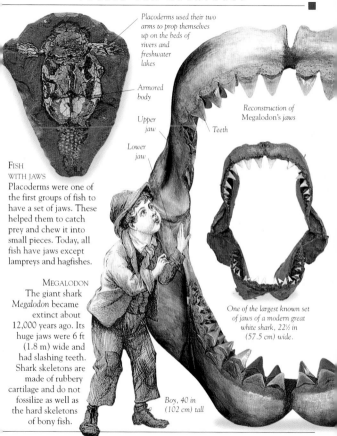

Placoderms used their two arms to prop themselves up on the beds of rivers and freshwater lakes

Armored body

Upper jaw

Lower jaw

Teeth

Reconstruction of Megalodon's jaws

FISH WITH JAWS

Placoderms were one of the first groups of fish to have a set of jaws. These helped them to catch prey and chew it into small pieces. Today, all fish have jaws except lampreys and hagfishes.

MEGALODON

The giant shark *Megalodon* became extinct about 12,000 years ago. Its huge jaws were 6 ft (1.8 m) wide and had slashing teeth. Shark skeletons are made of rubbery cartilage and do not fossilize as well as the hard skeletons of bony fish.

One of the largest known set of jaws of a modern great white shark, 22½ in (57.5 cm) wide.

Boy, 40 in (102 cm) tall

99

FOSSIL AMPHIBIANS AND REPTILES

EARLY AMPHIBIANS developed from fleshy-finned fish 380 million years ago. They were the first four-legged animals to walk on land. Reptiles, which could survive and reproduce away from water, evolved after amphibians. Finally, mammal-like reptiles gave rise to mammals.

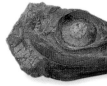

MARINE REPTILE
Ichthyosaurus, or "fish reptile," developed from a land-living reptile that adapted to life in the water. It had long jaws and short, sharp teeth for catching fish.

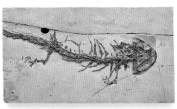

ANDRIAS
The skeleton of the extinct giant salamander *Andrias* was well designed for swimming, with a long, powerful tail. Some modern salamanders also reach a very large size – the Japanese giant salamander can grow to over 5 ft (1.5 m) long.

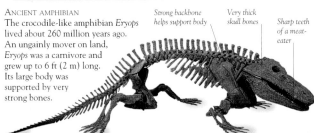

ANCIENT AMPHIBIAN
The crocodile-like amphibian *Eryops* lived about 260 million years ago. An ungainly mover on land, *Eryops* was a carnivore and grew up to 6 ft (2 m) long. Its large body was supported by very strong bones.

Strong backbone helps support body

Very thick skull bones

Sharp teeth of a meat-eater

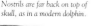

Nostrils are far back on top of skull, as in a modern dolphin.

Long snout

Short, sharp teeth

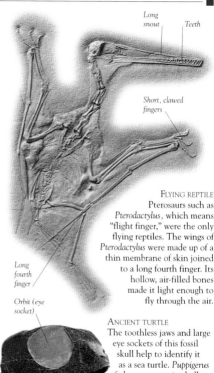

Long snout

Teeth

Short, clawed fingers

Long fourth finger

Orbit (eye socket)

Quadrate

Articular REPTILE SKULL

Quadrate

Articular CYNODONT SKULL

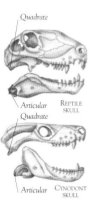

REPTILES LIKE MAMMALS
All mammals developed from the cynodonts, a single group of mammal-like reptiles. The quadrate and articular bones in the jaw hinges of cynodonts eventually developed into the three bones of the mammal ear.

FLYING REPTILE
Pterosaurs such as *Pterodactylus*, which means "flight finger," were the only flying reptiles. The wings of *Pterodactylus* were made up of a thin membrane of skin joined to a long fourth finger. Its hollow, air-filled bones made it light enough to fly through the air.

ANCIENT TURTLE
The toothless jaws and large eye sockets of this fossil skull help to identify it as a sea turtle. *Puppigerus* fed on sea grass in shallow coastal waters and had a smooth shell with many bony plates. *Puppigerus* lived about 40 million years ago.

Toothless jaws

DINOSAURS

FOR 150 MILLION YEARS, the Earth
was dominated by the dinosaurs,
a group of reptiles that died
out about 65 million years ago.

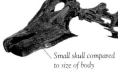

*Small skull compared
to size of body*

Dinosaurs lived on land and were unable to swim
or fly. They were also the only reptiles ever to walk
with straight legs directly under their bodies. Fossils
of whole dinosaur skeletons are very rare.

LIZARD HIPS AND BIRD HIPS

ORNITHISCHIAN PELVIS
Dinosaurs fall into two categories, based on
the arrangement of their pelvis (hipbones).
In ornithischian (bird-hipped) dinosaurs,
the pubis slanted back, parallel to the
backward-pointing ischium.
Dinosaurs in this
category were
plant-eaters.

Pubis

IGUANODON
(BIRD-HIPPED)

SAURISCHIAN PELVIS
In saurischian (lizard-hipped)
dinosaurs, the pubis
pointed downward
and forward, and the ischium
downward and backward.
Saurischians were either
plant- or meat-eaters.

Pubis

TYRANNOSAURUS REX
(LIZARD-HIPPED)

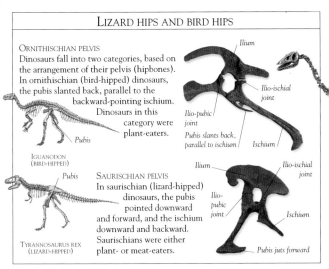

Ilium

*Ilio-ischial
joint*

*Ilio-pubic
joint*

*Pubis slants back,
parallel to ischium*

Ischium

Ilium

*Ilio-ischial
joint*

*Ilio-
pubic
joint*

Ischium

Pubis juts forward

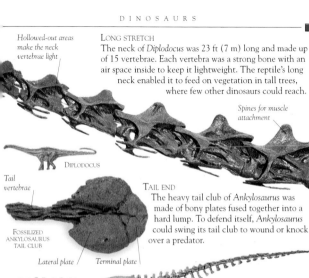

Hollowed-out areas make the neck vertebrae light

LONG STRETCH

The neck of *Diplodocus* was 23 ft (7 m) long and made up of 15 vertebrae. Each vertebra was a strong bone with an air space inside to keep it lightweight. The reptile's long neck enabled it to feed on vegetation in tall trees, where few other dinosaurs could reach.

Spines for muscle attachment

DIPLODOCUS

Tail vertebrae

TAIL END

The heavy tail club of *Ankylosaurus* was made of bony plates fused together into a hard lump. To defend itself, *Ankylosaurus* could swing its tail club to wound or knock over a predator.

FOSSILIZED ANKYLOSAURUS TAIL CLUB

Lateral plate   *Terminal plate*

Long tail provided balance when running at high speed

Fused foot bones formed lower part of leg

Only the toes of Struthiomimus touched the ground

FAST RUNNER

Struthiomimus, which means "ostrich mimic," had thin, powerful back legs built for sprinting, like a modern ostrich. Unlike an ostrich, it had mobile, clawed arms instead of wings, and a long, bony tail.

DINOSAUR FACTS

• The tallest dinosaur was *Ultrasaurus*. At 53–56 ft (16–17 m) tall, it was as high as a three story building.

• *Ankylosaurus* was the widest dinosaur – at 16½ ft (5 m) across it was similar in size and shape to an army tank.

• *Struthiomimus* could run faster than a horse.

Dinosaur skulls

The shape and size of a dinosaur's skull reveal a lot about how it lived. The jaws and teeth show whether a dinosaur was a plant-eater, a meat-eater, or had a varied diet. Horns were used for defense or attack, while head crests may have been used to attract mates or to warn others of approaching danger.

MASSOSPONDYLUS SKULL
The small, coarse-edged teeth of the early dinosaur *Massospondylus* were suitable for chewing both meat and plants. Animals that can feed in this way are called omnivores.

TYRANNOSAURUS REX TOOTH

Jagged edges for tearing flesh

Sharp edge of unworn tooth

Tooth worn down by diet of tough plants

IGUANODON TEETH

DINOSAUR TEETH
Some plant-eating (herbivorous) dinosaurs, such as *Iguanodon*, had grinding, crushing teeth for chewing tough, fibrous plants. Others, like *Triceratops*, were equipped with sharp, slicing teeth. A meat-eating (carnivorous) dinosaur, such as *Tyrannosaurus rex*, had rows of jagged teeth for cutting and tearing meat.

BRAIN CASTS
Dinosaur brains were too soft to fossilize, but casts from the inside of dinosaur skulls show us their different shapes and sizes. It is likely most dinosaurs were as intelligent as modern reptiles.

BAROSAURUS BRAIN CAST

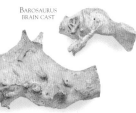

TYRANNOSAURUS REX BRAIN CAST

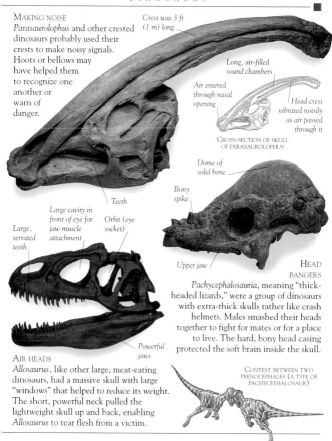

MAKING NOISE
Parasaurolophus and other crested dinosaurs probably used their crests to make noisy signals. Hoots or bellows may have helped them to recognize one another or warn of danger.

Crest was 3 ft (1 m) long

Long, air-filled sound chambers

Air entered through nasal opening

Head crest vibrated noisily as air passed through it

CROSS-SECTION OF SKULL OF PARASAUROLOPHUS

Dome of solid bone

Bony spike

Teeth

Large cavity in front of eye for jaw muscle attachment

Orbit (eye socket)

Large, serrated teeth

Upper jaw

Powerful jaws

HEAD BANGERS
Pachycephalosauria, meaning "thick-headed lizards," were a group of dinosaurs with extra-thick skulls rather like crash helmets. Males smashed their heads together to fight for mates or for a place to live. The hard, bony head casing protected the soft brain inside the skull.

AIR HEADS
Allosaurus, like other large, meat-eating dinosaurs, had a massive skull with large "windows" that helped to reduce its weight. The short, powerful neck pulled the lightweight skull up and back, enabling *Allosaurus* to tear flesh from a victim.

CONTEST BETWEEN TWO PRENOCEPHALES (A TYPE OF PACHYCEPHALOSAUR)

FOSSIL MAMMALS

WHEN DINOSAURS became extinct about 65 million years ago, mammal species became more varied and numerous. Pouched mammals (marsupials) were more widespread in prehistoric times, but placental mammals (where the young develop inside the mother's womb) are now dominant in most parts of the world.

Wide pelvis for leg muscle attachment

Foot

MEGAZOSTRODON
The early mammal *Megazostrodon* was rather like a modern shrew. Unlike scaly, cold-blooded reptiles, *Megazostrodon* was covered with body hair, which provided insulation, and could maintain a constant body temperature.

Pelvis

MEGAZOSTRODON

Epipubic (marsupial) bone

Chisel-like molar teeth

Bony horn with furrows left by blood vessels

Pillarlike legs to support weight

ARSINOITHERIUM
The massive horn of *Arsinoitherium*, an extinct rhinoceros-like mammal, was made of bone. In a modern rhinoceros, the horn is made from compressed hair. *Arsinoitherium's* chisel-edged molar teeth indicate that it fed mainly on leaves.

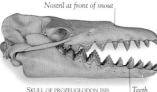

Nostril at front of snout

SKULL OF PROZEUGLODON ISIS | *Teeth*

PROZEUGLODON ISIS
Skulls of early whales show that the nostrils were originally at the front of the snout, but gradually moved back onto the top of the head. This change allowed a whale to breathe air at the the water's surface without having to lift its whole head out of the water.

High nasal bone

Blunt tooth for grinding vegetation

Rib cage

Curved incisor tooth

DIPROTODON
This stocky, short-limbed animal lived in Australia until about 10,000 years ago. At 10 ft (3 m) long, *Diprotodon* was one of the largest, plant-eating marsupials around, with blunt, plant-grinding cheek teeth and huge, rodentlike incisors. It is possible that *Diprotodon* was hunted by early humans.

DIPROTODON

THYLACOSMILUS
The extinct mammal *Thylacosmilus* was a marsupial that lived in South America about five million years ago. Although it closely resembled a placental saber-toothed tiger, it had no connection with the cat family.

Large heel bone

Long canine tooth

Bony tooth guard

HUMAN FOSSILS

THE EARLIEST human fossil remains date back five million years. By looking at the bones of early humans (hominids) it is possible to see how the size of the skull gradually increased to house a larger brain. The fossil remains also show how the pelvis shape changed to allow upright walking on two legs.

PROCONSUL SKULL

HOMO HEIDELBERGENSIS
This hominid lived in Africa and Asia about 500,000 years ago. *Homo heidelbergensis* may have given rise to two different species, *Homo neanderthalensis*, which is now extinct, and modern humans, *Homo sapiens*.

No forehead

Large brow (supraorbital) ridges

Large upper jaw

PROCONSUL AFRICANUS
One of the earliest apes, *Proconsul* lived about 18 million years ago in the woods and forests of modern-day Kenya. It had the long pelvis and arms of a monkey, but an apelike skull.

Backbone shape typical of a four-legged animal

AUSTRALOPITHECUS
The earliest known hominid, *Australopithecus afarensis*, was 3 ft 7 in (1.1 m) tall. Its strong leg bones, broad pelvis, and S-shaped backbone enabled it to walk upright on two legs.

Small cranium

Short, broad pelvis

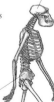

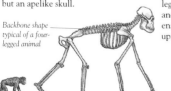

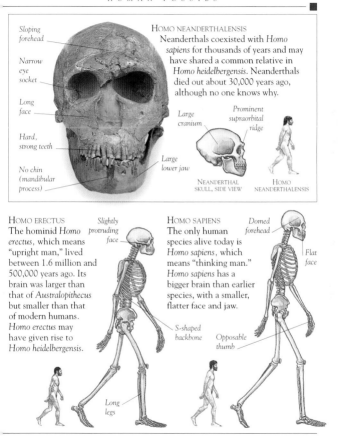

Sloping forehead

Narrow eye socket

Long face

Hard, strong teeth

No chin (mandibular process)

Large lower jaw

HOMO NEANDERTHALENSIS

Neanderthals coexisted with *Homo sapiens* for thousands of years and may have shared a common relative in *Homo heidelbergensis*. Neanderthals died out about 30,000 years ago, although no one knows why.

Large cranium

Prominent supraorbital ridge

NEANDERTHAL SKULL, SIDE VIEW

HOMO NEANDERTHALENSIS

HOMO ERECTUS

The hominid *Homo erectus*, which means "upright man," lived between 1.6 million and 500,000 years ago. Its brain was larger than that of *Australopithecus* but smaller than that of modern humans. *Homo erectus* may have given rise to *Homo heidelbergensis*.

Slightly protruding face

S-shaped backbone

Long legs

HOMO SAPIENS

The only human species alive today is *Homo sapiens*, which means "thinking man." *Homo sapiens* has a bigger brain than earlier species, with a smaller, flatter face and jaw.

Domed forehead

Flat face

Opposable thumb

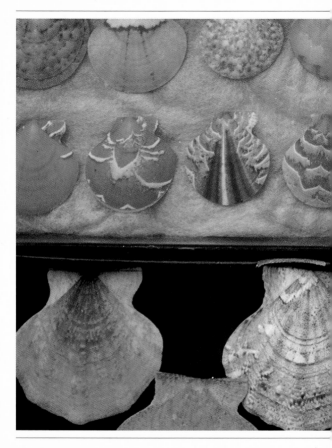

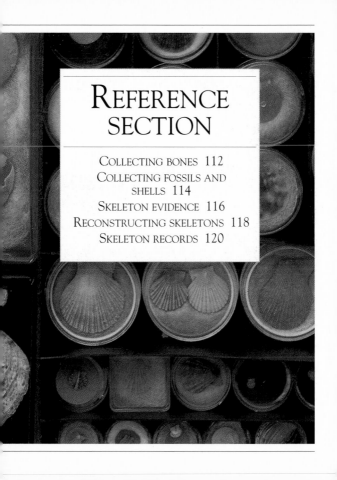

REFERENCE
SECTION

COLLECTING BONES

By COLLECTING and examining
bones, much can be learned
about the skeletons, methods
of feeding, and lifestyles of
vertebrates. Bones may be
found by roadsides, in gardens,
washed up on beaches, or as
leftovers from cooking, such
as fish or chicken bones.

Internal channels in bone are visible

Centrum

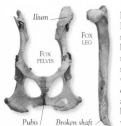

Ilium

FOX
LEG

FOX
PELVIS

Pubis *Broken shaft*

ROADSIDE CASUALTY
Foxes are often killed by
motor vehicles; these
bones were found near a
road. Recovered bones
should always be cleaned
with soapy water and
disinfectant. Remove
any remaining flesh by
boiling the bones in
water for two hours.

BEACH DEBRIS
This vertebra from
the backbone of a fur
seal was washed up on
the Skeleton Coast of
Namibia, southwest
Africa. The salty seawater
has dissolved away some
of the bone to reveal the
internal structure.

JAWS AND TEETH
Predators rarely eat the jaws and teeth
of their prey. Teeth, which are firmly
connected to the jawbone, are too
hard to grind up. An animal's jaws and
teeth provide clues about what it eats
(see pp. 24–25). The teeth and jaws
of small animals are sometimes found
when digging in the yard or may be
brought into the home by pet cats.

Carnassial tooth

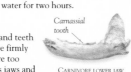

CARNIVORE LOWER JAW

Incisor tooth

RODENT LOWER JAW

Flat, grinding top

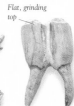

HERBIVORE'S TOOTH

OWL PELLETS

HIDDEN CONTENTS

Like many birds of prey, owls cough up indigestible parts of their food, such as bones, as tightly packed pellets. Look for these in the woods under trees where owls roost. To reveal their contents, soak the pellets in warm water for half an hour and then gently pull them apart with tweezers.

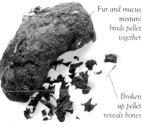

Fur and mucus mixture binds pellet together

Broken up pellet reveals bones

Skull

Ribs are curved with flattened sides

Orbit (eye socket)

Shoulder blades attach to front legs

VOLE BONES

Leg bones

BONE GROUPS

Sort the bones in each pellet into groups, such as skulls, limb bones, vertebrae, ribs, and shoulder bones. Try to identify which animals the bones come from. This pellet shows that the owl that produced it had dined exclusively on voles.

BIRD BONES

Owls feed mainly on rodents, such as voles, but these starling bones were found in a tawny owl pellet. This indicates that birds are also part of the owl's diet. The owl has managed to swallow and regurgitate the starling's large skull almost intact.

Upper beak

Orbit (eye socket)

Skull

Leg, with claws still attached

Lower half of beak

Claws are made of indigestible protein

STARLING BONES

1 1 3

COLLECTING FOSSILS AND SHELLS

BUILDING UP your own collection of fossils and shells can be an enjoyable pastime and helps with identifying and understanding skeletons. When looking for specimens, wear suitable clothes, and take the correct tools. Shells are usually found on beaches, while fossils are found inside rocks.

GLOVES

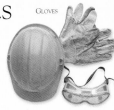

HARD HAT   GOGGLES

PROTECTIVE CLOTHING
When collecting fossils, wear gloves to protect your hands from sharp rocks. Goggles will keep dust and rock fragments out of your eyes. A hard hat is also essential to protect your head from falling rocks.

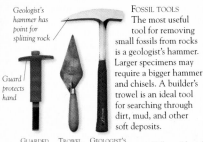

Geologist's hammer has point for splitting rock

Guard protects hand

GUARDED CHISEL   TROWEL   GEOLOGIST'S HAMMER

FOSSIL TOOLS
The most useful tool for removing small fossils from rocks is a geologist's hammer. Larger specimens may require a bigger hammer and chisels. A builder's trowel is an ideal tool for searching through dirt, mud, and other soft deposits.

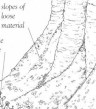

Beware of falling rocks from cliff top

Do not collect on unstable slopes of loose material

Collect safely at the bottom of the slope

Make sure that you are allowed to remove fossils.

FOSSIL HUNTING SITES
To find fossil-bearing sedimentary rocks, look up suitable sites on a geological map. Likely sites are areas where the rocks are exposed, such as cliffs, quarries, caves, and road cuttings.

CLEANING TOOLS
Wrap any fossil finds or shells in newspaper, and clean them carefully at home. Toothbrushes and tweezers are useful for removing mud, soil, and sand. A sharp knife, penknife, or chisel may also be needed to remove ingrained dirt, but take care not to damage the specimen.

TWEEZERS   TOOTHBRUSH   MAGNIFYING
GLASS

Use to
examine
details

CLEANING TECHNIQUES
When cleaning shells and fossils, it is important to be careful, gentle, and patient. Before washing, make sure that water will not damage the specimens. Do not brush or scrape the surface of fossil specimens preserved in chalk, as this will remove surface detail.

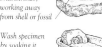

Use careful brushstrokes, working away from shell or fossil

Wash specimen by soaking it in a bath of warm water

STORING COLLECTIONS
Fossils and shells should be stored away from moisture and dust. Shells fade when exposed to light, so store them in the dark. Small cabinets with shallow drawers are ideal, and small boxes or glass tubes can be used to divide types within the drawers. Shoeboxes, matchboxes, and cabinets for screws and washers are also useful.

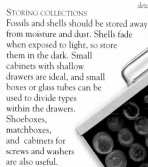
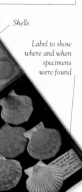

Shells

Label to show where and when specimens were found

Plastic boxes with identification labels

SKELETON EVIDENCE

HUMAN SKELETONS may be preserved by burial in tombs and coffins, or by natural causes, such as desert heat, extreme cold, or waterlogged soil. Some skeletons have been exceptionally well preserved by natural or artificial mummification. They provide valuable evidence of the health, lifestyle, and beliefs of people from ancient civilizations.

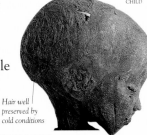

MUMMIFIED HEAD OF PERUVIAN CHILD

Lower jaw

Left orbit (eye socket)

Teeth

Hair well preserved by cold conditions

MUMMIFIED CHILD
This head belongs to a child from the ancient civilization at Arica, Peru (c. 5800–2000 BC). Buried as a result of an earthquake, the child's body was mummified by cold, arid conditions. Its age at death can be figured out by examining the skull sutures and teeth.

MUMMY'S SKULL
This X ray allows close examination of the skull without damaging the mummified remains. The erupting teeth in the lower jaw indicate that the child was two years old when it died.

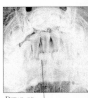

UNDERSIDE OF SKULL

DETAIL OF LOWER JAW

Erupting teeth

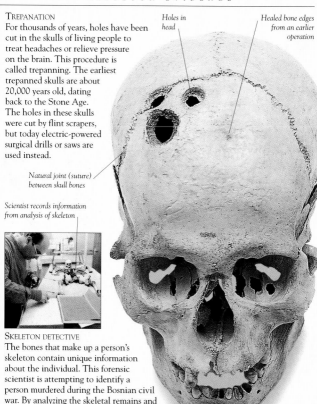

TREPANATION

For thousands of years, holes have been cut in the skulls of living people to treat headaches or relieve pressure on the brain. This procedure is called trepanning. The earliest trepanned skulls are about 20,000 years old, dating back to the Stone Age. The holes in these skulls were cut by flint scrapers, but today electric-powered surgical drills or saws are used instead.

Holes in head

Healed bone edges from an earlier operation

Natural joint (suture) between skull bones

Scientist records information from analysis of skeleton

SKELETON DETECTIVE

The bones that make up a person's skeleton contain unique information about the individual. This forensic scientist is attempting to identify a person murdered during the Bosnian civil war. By analyzing the skeletal remains and checking them against medical records, the dead individual may eventually be identified.

PRESERVED
SKULL
C. 2000 BC

RECONSTRUCTING SKELETONS

WHEN THE SKELETONS of long-dead humans or animals are discovered, they are usually found broken into pieces. Complete skeletons are carefully dismantled and taken to a museum or laboratory. Using their knowledge of anatomy to study the bones, scientists can reconstruct both the skeleton and the physical appearance of its owner.

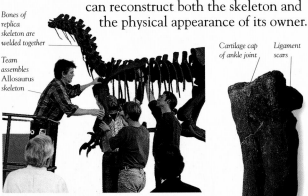

Bones of replica skeleton are welded together

Team assembles Allosaurus skeleton

Cartilage cap of ankle joint

Ligament scars

MUSEUM PIECE
Most of the big, mounted dinosaur skeletons on display in museums today are replicas of the originals. Made of lightweight plastic and fiberglass, they are supported by a framework of thin metal rods. The original fossil bones were so heavy that they had to be supported by scaffolding.

CLUES FROM THE BONE
Ligament scars along the length of this *Iguandon* foot bone indicate where muscles and other bones were attached when the dinosaur was alive. Rough surfaces on the bone ends mark the attachment points of ankle and toe joint cartilage.

Cartilage surface of joint for toe

RECONSTRUCTING A DINOSAUR

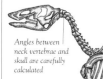

Angles between neck vertebrae and skull are carefully calculated

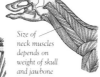

Size of neck muscles depends on weight of skull and jawbone

Skin forms a protective covering over muscles

1 BONY JIGSAW
First, the bones are fitted together. Model replicas of any missing bones are made using fiberglass or plastic. The skeleton is then ready to be fleshed out.

2 MUSCLE ATTACHMENT
The size and shape of a dinosaur's muscles can be calculated by looking at the attachment scars on its bones. Studying modern reptile anatomy also aids reconstruction.

3 REPTILE SKIN
Finally the skin is added. Impressions of dinosaur skin are sometimes preserved as fossils, but the color is a matter of guesswork based on living reptiles.

RECONSTRUCTING FACES
The face of a person who lived thousands of years ago can be recreated by building up a clay face on top of a replica of their skull. Pegs mark key points on the skull where the thickness of soft tissues is known. Muscles are then added in clay, with extra material to represent fat, nerves, and blood vessels. The size and shape of ears and mouths is largely guesswork.

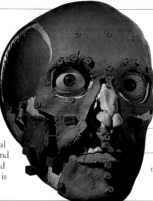

Eye color, skin condition, and color of hair must be guessed

Shape of nose cartilage depends on skull's shape

Marking peg

Reconstructed face belongs to the Ice Man, who died in the Alps 4,000 years ago

SKELETON RECORDS

ANIMAL SKELETONS vary in size and shape, but they all provide support, protection, and mobility. Some parts of a skeleton can be tiny, while others may grow to huge proportions. Here are some of the more amazing examples.

HUMAN SKELETON

Longest, strongest bone
The femur (thighbone) is about one-quarter of a person's height and can withstand a weight of over a ton (metric ton).

Smallest human bone
The tiny stapes (stirrup bone) in the ear is about ⅛ in (3 mm) long.

Tallest skeleton
The tallest recorded skeleton belonged to Robert Pershing Wadlow, USA, who grew to 8 ft 10 in (2.7 m) tall.

Joint records
The largest joint is the knee, which connects the upper and lower leg bones.

Smallest skeletons
The smallest humans have skeletons that grow to a height of about 2½ ft (60–75 cm).

FEMUR

SKELETONS ON THE INSIDE

Longest bony fish
The long, internal skeleton of an oarfish can reach a length of nearly 50 ft (15.2 m).

Smallest bird skeleton
The tiny skeleton of the male bee hummingbird grows to about 2¼ in (5.7 cm) in length.

AUSTRALIAN PELICAN

Longest bird bill
The bill of the Australian pelican may grow up to 1½ ft (47 cm) long.

Largest endoskeleton
The blue whale has the largest endoskeleton of any living animal, measuring about 110 ft (33.5 m) in length.

Largest reptile skeleton
The saltwater crocodile's endoskeleton can reach a length of 33 ft (10 m).

SKELETONS ON THE OUTSIDE

Largest crustacean
The exoskeleton of the Japanese spider crab can reach a width of up to 13 ft (4 m) across the span of its claws.

Smallest crustacean
The outer shell of the Alonella flea is as tiny as a grain of salt.

Longest insect skeleton
The giant stick insect of Borneo has an exoskeleton measuring up to 20 in (50 cm) long.

Largest sea urchin shell
The Japanese sea urchin *Sperosoma giganteum* has a shell diameter of 12½ in (32 cm).

Largest arachnid skeleton
The exoskeleton of the southern Indian scorpion *Heterometrus swannerdami* grows to over 7 in (18 cm) in length.

Largest shellfish
The shell of the giant clam can reach a width of 39 in (1 m) across.

Largest spider skeleton
The exoskeleton of the huge Goliath bird-eating spider from South America can reach a width of up to 11 in (28 cm) across the span of its legs.

JAPANESE SPIDER CRAB

ANCIENT SKELETONS

Largest fossil antlers
The extinct Irish elk had the largest antlers ever recorded, measuring 14 ft (4.3 m) across.

Longest fossil teeth
The longest recorded fossil teeth belonged to *Tyrannosaurus rex*. Some of them measure up to 7 in (18 cm) long.

Longest fossil neck
The neck of the dinosaur *Mamenchisaurus* grew to a length of 33 ft (10 m).

Largest fossil insect
The largest prehistoric insect on record is the 300-million-year-old dragonfly *Meganeura monyi*. Its wings could grow to a span of up to 29½ in (75 cm).

Largest fossil bird
The wing bones of *Argentavis magnificens* spanned 25 ft (7.6 m).

Tallest dinosaur skeleton
The sauropod dinosaur *Brachiosaurus* grew to a height of 39 ft (12 m).

IRISH ELK SKULL

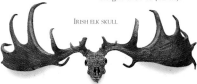

Glossary

AMPHIBIAN
A vertebrate that lives in water and on land, such as a frog or newt.

ARACHNID
An arthropod with four pairs of walking legs, such as a spider, tick, or scorpion.

ARTHROPOD
An invertebrate with a segmented body, jointed legs, and an exoskeleton. The arthropod group includes crustaceans, arachnids, and insects.

CAMOUFLAGE
To blend in with the surroundings to hide from predators and prey.

CANINE TOOTH
A pointed tooth next to the incisors that grips and pierces prey.

CARNASSIAL TOOTH
A shearing tooth of a carnivore. Upper-jaw carnassial teeth are formed from the last premolars. Lower-jaw carnassials are formed from the first molars.

CARNIVORE
A meat-eating animal.

CARPAL
Vertebrate wrist bone.

CARTILAGE
A tough, slippery substance in a vertebrate skeleton that protects the joints. Cartilaginous fish (sharks and rays) have a skeleton made of cartilage.

CHITIN
A light, strong, substance found in the exoskeletons of arthropods.

COLLAGEN
A structural protein found in bone and tissues that forms strong, elastic fibers.

CRANIUM
The part of the skull surrounding the brain.

CRUSTACEAN
A group of mainly aquatic arthropods, typically with a hard case, or "crust," that encloses the body.

DENTINE
Hard substance, also called ivory, found beneath the enamel of vertebrate teeth.

ECHINODERM
A marine invertebrate, with a skeleton formed from hard, bony plates called ossicles.

ENAMEL
A tough substance that forms the outer coating of vertebrate teeth.

ENDOSKELETON
A hard skeleton located inside an animal's body.

EXOSKELETON
A shell or hard skeleton on the outside of an animal's body.

FEMUR
Vertebrate thighbone.

FORENSIC SCIENCE
The analysis of skeletal or biological material in regard to questions of civil or criminal law.

GEOLOGY
The scientific study of the Earth's physical history and the rocks from which the planet is composed.

HERBIVORE
A plant-eating animal.

HOMINID
A family of primates that includes humans and their direct ancestors.

HYDROSTATIC SKELETON
A type of invertebrate skeleton maintained by the internal pressure of body fluids.

INCISOR TOOTH
A chisel-shaped cutting tooth at the front of the mouth in vertebrates.

INVERTEBRATE
An animal without a backbone.

KERATIN
A structural protein that forms strong, flexible fibers and makes up horn, hair, and nails.

LIGAMENT
A strong, fibrous band of tissue that joins bones together at joints.

MANDIBLE
A vertebrate's lower jaw, or the biting mouthpart of an arthropod.

MARROW
A substance found in spongy bone that makes red blood cells.

MAXILLA
Vertebrate upper jaw, or arthropod mouthpart to rear of the mandible.

MOLAR TOOTH
Chewing tooth at the side of a vertebrate jaw.

MOLLUSK
An invertebrate with a soft body, typically covered by a hard shell. The group includes snails and clams.

MOLT
The periodic shedding of an outer covering to allow for growth and renewal.

MUMMIFICATION
The process of drying and preserving either human or animal remains, by natural or artficial means.

NOCTURNAL
Occurring only at night.

OMNIVORE
An animal that eats both plants and other animals.

ORBIT
A bony socket in which the eyeball is situated.

OSSICLE
Any small bone or other calcified structure, such as a plate of an echinoderm shell or exoskeleton.

PHALANGES
The bones of the fingers or toes in vertebrates.

PREMOLAR TOOTH
Vertebrate tooth situated in front of the molars.

PRONOTUM
Protective head shield in some insect exoskeletons.

REPTILE
A vertebrate with scaly skin that lays sealed eggs, such as a chameleon, snake, lizard, crocodile, or tortoise.

RODENT
A small mammal with continuously growing, gnawing incisors.

SAUROPOD
A large, herbivorous dinosaur that walked on all fours, with a long neck and tail and a small head.

SCAPULA
Vertebrate shoulder blade.

SEDIMENT
Mineral or organic matter carried and deposited by water, wind, or ice.

SEDIMENTARY ROCK
Rock formed from layers of sediment.

SPINAL CORD
The cord of nerve tissue enclosed and protected by the spinal column.

STERNUM
Vertebrate breastbone.

TARSAL
Vertebrate anklebone.

TUSK
A vertebrate tooth that projects beyond the upper or lower jaw.

VERTEBRA
A bone that forms part of the spinal column.

VERTEBRATE
An animal with a bony or cartilaginous spinal column (backbone).

Index

Acknowledgments

PAGEOne and DK Publishing would like to thank:
Hilary Bird for compiling the index, Marcus James and Jane Yorke at Dorling Kindersley Ltd., and Dean Price for the jacket design.

Illustrations by:
David Ashby, Joanna Cameron, Martin Camm, Giuliano Fornari, Will Giles, Mark Iley, Alan Jackson, Kenneth Lilly, Andrew Macdonald, Debbie Maizels, Sandra Pond, Graham Rosewarne, John Temperton, Simon Thomas, Peter Visscher, Andrew Williams, John Woodcock.

Photographs by:
Peter Anderson, Geoff Brightling, Jane Burton, Peter Chadwick, Tina Chambers, Andy Crawford, Geoff Dann, Richard Davies, Phillip Dowell, John Downes, Andreas von Einsiedel, Neil Fletcher, Lynton Gardiner, Steve Gorton, Trevor Graham, Frank Greenaway, Colin Keates, Barnabas Kindersley, Dave King, Tracy Morgan, Roger Phillips, Tim Ridley, Karl Shone, Clive Streeter, Harry Taylor, Kim Taylor, Matthew Ward.

Picture credits:
t=top b=bottom c=center l=left r=right
AKG Photo 48br; Bodleian Library 59tr; Bridgeman Art Library 40br; Bruce Coleman Ltd./Alain Compost 74tr, John Shaw 23tl; Kenneth Garrett Photography 119b; Frank Lane Picture Agency/David Hosking 73tl; Natural History Museum 16r, 23r, 24b, 24cr, 25c, 26bl, 26br, 30cr, 31tc, 31tl, 32r, 37cb, 71c, 72br, 72cb, 106bl, 106–107, 108cr, 108tl, 109tl, 120r, 121b; Oxford Scientific Films/Mark Deeble and Victoria Stone 12cl, Daniel J. Fox 65br, Michele Hall 86t, Survival Anglia, Des and Jen Bartlett 68cr; Oxford University Museum 12–13, 35l, 56tr; Planet Earth Pictures/Beth Davidow 29l, Larry Tackett 30br; Rex Features/Damir, SIPA Press 117l; Royal Veterinary College 61br; Science Photo Library/Chris Bjornberg 51l, Scott Camazine 16l, CNRI 21bl, Jan Hinsch 17br, Dr Morley Read 92l, Prof P. Mott, Dept of Anatomy, University La Sapienza, Rome 18tr, 19tl, J. C. Revy 47bl; Smithsonian Institute 99r; The Stock Market/Damm 46tl; University Museum of Zoology, Cambridge 28cl; Jerry Young 90bc.

Every effort has been made to trace the copyright holders and we apologize in advance for any unintentional omissions. We would be pleased to insert the appropriate acknowledgment in any subsequent edition of this publication.